LYING AND DECEPTION IN EVERYDAY LIFE

Lying and Deception
in
Everyday Life

MICHAEL LEWIS
CAROLYN SAARNI
Editors

THE GUILFORD PRESS
New York   London

© 1993 The Guilford Press
A Division of Guilford Publications, Inc.
72 Spring Street, New York, N. Y. 10012

Printed in the United States of America

This book is printed on acid-free paper

Last digit is print number: 9 8 7 6 5 4 3 2 1

Library of Congress Cataloging-in-Publication Data

Lewis, Michael, 1937, Jan. 10–
  Lying and deception in everyday life / Michael Lewis,
Carolyn Saarni.
    p.   cm.
  Includes bibliographical references and index.
  ISBN 0-89862-894-6
    1. Deception.   2. Self-deception.   3. Truthfulness and
falsehood.   I. Saarni, Carolyn.   II. Title.
  BF637.D42L49 1993
  177'.3—dc20   92-36145
                                                      CIP

Preface

Any interest in emotional life must lead one to question the relation between the outward social expression of emotion and the inward private world of our feelings. The discrepancy between our social smiling and "Oh, yes, thank you for your lovely gift" and the inward feeling of "Oh, how ugly!" must lead us to the topic of how people deceive.

While parents often observe deception in their children, and adults know of their own deception as well as that of others, it is impressive how resourceful people are when it comes to figuring out how to avoid feeling badly. Whether it be covering up one's misdeeds so as to avoid getting into trouble, masking how one expresses one's emotions, or repressing the genuine painfulness of stressful events in order to cope with them, people show considerable aptitude for deception.

The different views attending deception imply a dilemma that pits falsification against truth. At the individual level, this dilemma is resolved by "choosing" between them although it appears that we all use and need deception in order to cope with social life, both within ourselves and in our relationships with others.

The polarity between deception and truth has been discussed in disciplines as diverse as philosophy, psychology, sociology, theology, anthropology, and ethology. In order to address "lying and deception in everyday life," we desired to include contributors from several disciplines in order to explore the dimensions of deception. Because of the diverse perspectives, we asked that the contributors write with an eye to a readership that is similarly interdisciplinary in its interests.

We also wanted to explore the view that, given the ubiquity, the sheer ordinariness of deception, perhaps it was time to examine duplicity, not as the bane of existence, but rather as another example of how remarkably resourceful people are in their adaptation to the demands of living with others. This adaptiveness means they will use deception functionally and strategically, for both socially approved goals and for reasons that provoke distrust and condemnation.

We thought it also imperative to articulate the boundaries between deception that is unethical and deception that is adaptive. Our current political situation is mired down in trying to figure out such boundaries from a legalistic standpoint, and we think social scientists, philosophers, and clinicians have much to offer in clarifying what these boundaries may be and what functions are played by different sorts of deception.

Also cutting across most of the topics appearing in *Lying and Deception in Everyday Life* is the theme of emotion in human experience. Emotion, common to all humans, seems to be at the foundation of lying in everyday life. Topics such as how we learn to put on emotional "false fronts" and why we deceive ourselves are directly concerned with feelings, especially feelings that people have about themselves. We think this focus on emotion sets *Lying and Deception in Everyday Life* apart from other books on deception. It most certainly humanizes the topic of deception and diminishes the near-taboo quality often associated with investigations of deceit.

MICHAEL LEWIS
CAROLYN SAARNI

List of Contributors

Roy F. Baumeister, PhD, Department of Psychology, Case Western Reserve University, Cleveland, Ohio

Bella DePaulo, PhD, Department of Psychology, University of Virginia, Charlottesville, Virginia

Paul Ekman, PhD, Department of Psychiatry, University of California, San Francisco, California

Jennifer A. Epstein, PhD, Department of Psychology, University of Virginia, Charlottesville, Virginia

Mark G. Frank, PhD, Department of Psychiatry, University of California, San Francisco, California

P. Randall Kropp, PhD, Director of Research, British Columbia Institute on Family Violence, Vancouver, British Coumbia, Canada

Michael Lewis, PhD, Department of Pediatrics, UMDNJ—Robert Wood Johnson Medical School, New Brunswick, New Jersey.

Robert Mitchell, PhD, Department of Psychology, Eastern Kentucky University, Richmond, Kentucky

Richard Rogers, PhD, Department of Psychology, University of North Texas, Denton, Texas

Carolyn Saarni, PhD, Department of Counseling, Sonoma State University, Rohnert Park, California

C. R. Snyder, PhD, Department of Psychology, University of Kansas, Lawrence, Kansas

Sandra Tate Sigmon, PhD, Department of Psychology, University of Maine, Orono, Maine

Robert C. Solomon, PhD, Department of Philosophy, The University of Texas at Austin, Austin, Texas

Maria von Salisch, PhD, Free University of Berlin, Germany

Melissa M. Wyer, PhD, Department of Psychology, University of Virginia, Charlottesville, Virginia

Contents

1
Deceit and Illusion in Human Affairs

CAROLYN SAARNI
MICHAEL LEWIS

As editors, we have thought hard about how best to inform readers about what to expect in this volume. As we have contemplated lying and deception in everyday life, we have not recoiled at the presumed moral turpitude of it all; rather we have looked with some compassion at how intricately people construct lies and illusions in their lives. If deception is so pervasive in our culture, what fuels it? Other questions that have intrigued us include whether some kinds of deception may be unconscious. Does this mean that we are not responsible for the consequences of such lies? Might the need for illusions about oneself fall into such a category of deception? Why does self-deception or the need for illusion make us feel uncomfortable? There appears to be considerable emotion behind lying and deception, and perhaps it is the ubiquity of human feeling, emotions felt about ourselves and our relations with others, that motivates lying and deception and contributes to the latter's pervasiveness.

We shall give some "flesh and blood" to these questions of deception as well as introduce some of the issues taken up by the contributors to this volume on deception by presenting a script that includes many examples of lying. Think of it as similar to what television producers might work with as they try to imagine how effective it might be as a televised vignette. We shall asterisk some of the lies and deceptions. Can you find more examples?

A DAY IN THE LIFE OF ORDINARY PEOPLE

Scene 1

SETTING: It is 6:30 AM in Jan's and Ron's bedroom. The radio has just turned on. No one turns off the alarm or stirs, but Ron's blankets are in a heap while Jan's are neatly drawn up to her chin.

JAN: [*Camera zooms onto her face.*] Her eyes flick open toward the alarm clock and close again; her eyebrows knit together as in irritation and she pulls the blankets over her more tightly. A voice-over begins:

VOICE-OVER: "He always thinks I should turn off the alarm, because if I complain about how hard it is for me to wake up in the morning, then all the more reason I should throw myself out of bed like some kind of automaton. Well, I guess I'll just have to sleep soundly. . . ."*

RON: [*Camera zooms onto his face.*] A frown passes over his face.

VOICE-OVER: "She really ought to push herself to get up and turn that damn thing off. As usual, I have to do everything around here." [*Camera backs off.*] Ron staggers up, shuts it off, and leaves for the bathroom. Now in front of the mirror, he examines his face, widening his eyes, and baring his teeth.

VOICE-OVER: "Handsome devil, you. You're not god's gift to women, but you've been appreciated by quite a few [*smiles an exaggerated lecherous smile*], if I say so myself. I wish she did more of that appreciating [*jerks head toward bedroom*]. I could use some appreciating on another level from the 'Honcho' himself at work [*grimaces*]. He always wants more done, preferably all ready yesterday or even before he gives the order. As though we could all read his mind—if he has a mind. I wonder if Sharon is going to come by today [*smiles again*]. Now I sure could do some appreciating of her!"

JAN: [*Camera shows her now sprawled across the middle of the bed, a slight smile on her face, eyes still closed.*]

VOICE-OVER: "How delicious these extra five minutes in bed are! These few minutes are about the only time I get to myself it seems, that's why I need them—I don't control anything around here! Not that he would understand; he thinks I spend the day watching television or curling my hair. No appreciation for what goes into taking care of two kids and being a freelancer, not to speak of taking care of him too. Let's see, what's my mental priority list for today . . . ."

RON: [*Sticks head around side of bathroom door.*] "Jan, get up! Is this one of those mornings, again, where you need coffee first, in bed, before you can deal with the world?"

JAN: "As a matter of fact, I think it is one of those mornings. Thanks in advance, honey"* [*said in a sweet tone of voice with just a hint of saccharin*]. [*Pulls blankets up tightly around her again.*] "The girls will be in on top of me any minute now" [*pulls blanket all the way over her face*].

[*Background noise of young girls' voices and running feet. Camera switches to Ron in the kitchen pouring coffee with audible background evidence of the girls jumping on their mother and mutual happy morning greetings being exchanged.*]

RON: [*With a resigned facial expression.*]

VOICE-OVER: "Gotta put Sharon out of my mind. I love those girls, and I wouldn't want to break up this family for the world."

Scene 2

SETTING: Jan is on her way to an appointment at a magazine publisher's office; she uses the automatic change machine in the subway station in order to buy her ticket. Much to her obvious expressive pleasure, the machine dumps a huge handful of quarters, instead of the four that it should have, in exchange for her dollar bill. The money even spills out on the floor in front of the machine, making an attention-drawing clatter, as Jan scrambles to collect it all. Other passersby approach Jan.

JAN: "I just dropped my coin purse.* What a way to start the day! Sorry for the noise" [*smiles broadly at the two people closest to her*]. Jan hurriedly leaves the area.

Scene 3

SETTING: Ron is at work, and at the moment he is standing in the doorway to the office supply storage room with Sharon. They interact warmly: many smiles, head tilts, considerable eye contact, responsive body posture, etc.

RON: "How old did you say your son was, Sharon?"

SHARON: "He's 7 now; wait, I have a snapshot of him here [*digs in handbag and fishes it out*]. He's a real dear one, but awfully sensitive at times, you know, like he'll come home all upset over something some kid said to him. I guess he needs to develop a little more of a thick skin so he won't be so vulnerable. On the other hand, god forbid he should be like his father! His 'skin' was so thick, it was like steel, and just as cold too, inside and out!"

RON: "Must be hard being a single parent: Everything is your problem."

SHARON: "Yeah, but at least all I have is a kid to take care of and not a husband too."

RON: "Well, I take care of my wife, like bringing her coffee in bed in the mornings, and other things. I'm a feminist, you know [*said coyly*]."*

SHARON: "Hmmm, I've never met a man who said he was a feminist unless he had some strategy in mind [*said while looking sideways at Ron*]."

RON: "Oh, don't misunderstand me! What I mean is that I believe in equal rights for men and women, equal pay, and all that sort of thing."

SHARON: "Who does the laundry in your family?"

RON: [*Backing away a bit from Sharon.*] "My wife does. Look, I didn't come to argue with you" [*irritation flickers across his face but is quickly replaced with a contrite look;* then Ron brightens and changes the subject*]. "What do you think the Honcho is going to perpetrate on us at the next meeting?"

[*Camera switches to viewing Ron and Sharon walking down hallway, backs to the camera, a distinct distance between them. Then the camera zooms in on Ron, alone and appearing disgruntled, looking out the window from his office.*]

RON VOICE-OVER: "Did I blow it or did I blow it? But she's not worth the hassle.* In fact, I'll bet she even kind of enjoyed needling me about that laundry thing. Toxic woman, that's what. Good thing I'm a family man and have my values clear."*

Scene 4

SETTING: A board meeting at the advertising agency where Ron and Sharon both work; presiding is Mr. Lyecourt, otherwise known as the Honcho. The topic is an evaluation of how successful certain kinds of ad strategies are for selling a product.

SHARON: [*Alternately looking serious when turned toward her co-workers and smiling artfully when addressing the Honcho.*] "Our television perfume ads were designed to subtly arouse, and while viewers were in that aroused state, to design messages that would suggest they would be as sexually alluring as the model wearing the perfume.* We think it worked: compared to their levels before the ads started in the targeted area, sales of 'Compulsion' and 'Essence of Me' more than doubled. Our market survey revealed that the profile of the typical buyer was female, worked outside the home, watched television most evenings, and considered shopping a pleasurable pastime." [*She sits back in her chair and directs a confident smile around the room.*]

MR. LYECOURT: [*Initially looks approvingly at Sharon but then furrows his brow as he contemplates the remaining ad executives.*] "So, why don't the rest of you learn to do the same! You've got to figure out how to hit the viewers where they feel it: in their groin, their pocketbook, their looks, their status; what they mean to other people in their lives. The worst thing a person can feel is that he's trivial, meaningless, a bit of mold on a wall that can be washed off with a flick of a rag. Next to feeling this bad is just feeling ordinary. Now that's a lot more common, but people don't like to admit it: that they're ordinary. They always need to feel they're somehow special, whether it's their sex appeal, their brains, or their muscles. So go for it! Design ads that persuade people how to surpass ordinariness. That's what sells. After all, it's the American way, you know—the rugged individualist is ultimately a celebrity, because he's *special*, and you know how everyone wants their claim to fame." [*He sits back pompously and with an assurance that he's right.*]

Scene 5

SETTING: Jan sits hunched in front of her computer in a cramped, makeshift home office. She stares blankly ahead, and the screen on her monitor is also noticeably blank.

JAN VOICE-OVER: "I know I've got the ideas; they're hiding today or something. I have to keep reminding myself to be true to my own creativity and not get sucked into writing schlock, although it would be nice to make some money. There's so much trash out there that people are just dishing out because it's what sells or because it's what you have to do to get some recognition. Murder, mayhem, wild sex, child abuse, and international drug cartels—that's what's in nowadays. Oh, and let's not forget visions of Elvis and how to lose 50 pounds by going on an all-chocolate diet." [*Telephone rings in the background; Jan sighs and lets the answering machine respond, but she jumps up with alacrity, coffee flying all over her keyboard, and runs to the phone when she hears who is speaking on the other end.*]
     "Why, hello, Edna. I was just in the middle of something rather demanding and couldn't get to the phone right away* . . . So you're looking for something on extramarital sex and the lies that people tell about it . . . They would only pay $1500, hmmm . . . When would it be due? Well, that would be kind of rushing it. Hang on, let me check my calendar here* . . . Yes, I could do it, but I want an additional week . . . Yeah, I have a major project I'm trying to finish up* . . . No, I'd rather not reveal what it's about because I'm in the middle of some delicate

negotiations around it* . . . Glad you understand . . . Yeah, I know being an agent is tough stuff . . . Ok, send me the paperwork on it . . . ."

[A couple of minutes later, Jan phones up Ron at work.] "Hey, guess what! I got a real juicy assignment . . . Ha-ha, you'll never guess what it's on . . . This could be a real breakthrough for me, like I think this topic will really get noticed and get me some more contracts . . . No, I don't mind writing about this at all;* hey, it's what sells and gets a writer a little name recognition, sort of like your job, advertising."

Scene 6

SETTING: It's evening: Ron is looking at television and Jan is paying bills. Their daughters, 7-year-old Phoebe and 9-year-old Kate, are sprawled on the floor in the family room playing a board game and also involved in some kind of dispute.

KATE: [Looking disdainfully at her younger sister] "You are such a big baby, Phoebe, you always cry when you lose. You're no fun to play with!"

PHOEBE: [Looking distressed] "But you always beat me; I think you're a cheater!"

KATE: "No, I'm not; you're just dumb."

RON: "Kate, that really is out of bounds. I want you to apologize to Phoebe RIGHT NOW! And, Phoebe, you can't take these games so seriously; losers don't cry, they just grin and bear it and think about how to outfox the other player next time.* Ok, Kate, let's hear the apology."

KATE: [Averting her face from her father's view and looking quite contemptuously at her sister.] "Sorry."*

JAN: [Noticing Kate's facial expression toward her sister and her decidedly unenthusiastic tone of voice.] "Kate, do it again and this time mean it!"

KATE: [Adopting the briefest of thin-lipped smiles and a somewhat high-pitched tone of voice] "Sorry."

RON: "That's better. Why don't you guys get out your paints and I'll join you as soon as this program is over. By the way, Jan, that Sharon really alienated everyone today at our department meeting with old Lyecourt. Boy, she can be really underhanded."

JAN: "I thought you liked her and thought she was a really good addition to the group."

RON: "Guess it was just a first impression: Manipulation comes in all kinds of packages. Now, if I had a team-player like you, I'd be flying high at work!"*

JAN: "Why, Ron, that's really sweet of you to say that!"

[*The scene fades out and the television producer wonders what to do with the script. She files it away under the old soap opera series, "As the World Turns," and mutters to herself, "It's all so predictable."*]

FEELINGS AND DECEPTION

What we embedded in the preceding "predictable script" were the sorts of lies, illusions, and dissemblances that are commonly encountered in North American culture. Television family sitcoms are indeed a mirror to the kinds of deceptions we practice, often quite habitually, in our society. We apparently need illusions to feel good about ourselves and to maintain a sense of self-continuity. We lie to others in order to comfort them or protect their emotional well-being, as is the case in many "white" lies, or to mislead them as to our motives or our misdeeds, which would cause them anger and lead to our rejection or punishment. In our opinion, strong emotions are ultimately at the bottom of deception, for invariably emotion precedes lying and even more subtle forms of deception (as in having illusions about oneself or about one's close relationships): We *feel* ashamed when our self-esteem flags, because our illusions about ourselves are punctured and reality reveals our ordinariness or our failures. We *feel* afraid about being found out about a misdeed. We *feel* threatened by another's dominance or power over us and so perpetrate distortions to others to shore up our own insecurity and to damage the well-being of the dominant other. We *feel* envy or greed and want to possess that which a rival has, whether it be a stronger final quarter's earnings or romantic attention.

But we also *feel* caring and protective when we are aware that we have knowledge that could hurt someone we care about, and so we conceal from children the ugliness of what really went on behind the divorce. We *feel* concern and thus inhibit our disappointment, for example, at our spouse's ill-chosen but well intended gift, or feign pleasure with an aging parent upon agreeing once again to accompany him/her to the local Bingo game. We *feel* sympathy for the unfortunate, even as we also struggle with feeling aghast at their circumstances, such as when we encounter accident victims and attempt to conceal our expression of horror at their injuries. These kinds of feelings and our attempt to hide them are rampant, not only in our culture but in others as well.

And so we have it both ways: deception and lying can stem from emotions that lead us to be self-serving or from emotions that motivate us to be supportive and caring toward others. And the same individual is capable of both!

TAXONOMY OF LYING

In constructing a taxonomy of lies, there are many systems we might use for the many different kinds of lies. We lie about our feelings, we lie about what happened to us, we lie about what we want, we lie about what we are going to do. In some sense, then, deception and lying can occur in our every action, thought, and feeling. Lies, and the truth, occur much the same way as do the other opposites of our lives: hard and soft, loud and quiet, wet and dry. These opposites surround us and make the meaning of each member of the pair clearer. This, of course, is equally true for lying and truth telling. If we think about it for a moment, it is quite clear that the notion of something being true or truthful implies that there exist falseness and lies. We see no reason for ever doubting that anything is other than it appears if our minds were not also so constructed to believe that much of what we experience in others, in ourselves, and in the world around us is not true but false. In some profound sense, human experience has led to our belief that deception exists; that deception is part of the world around us. The search for truth as in knowing, the search for beauty, and even our religious quests all seem to center around the compelling desire to find the essence or core of reality. Part of our aesthetic, moral, religious, and intellectual struggles are designed to tear away deception and falsehood and to arrive at truth, at a state of grace with the world.

We would argue that deception, lying, falsehood, and masking of our inner selves exist as part of the social world in which we live. Because of this, the newborn child cannot help but be influenced by it. The child quickly comes to understand its existence, learns its rules, and becomes a very part of this process. Children, as well as adults, are immersed in interpersonal relationships and in relationships with the world, both of which have as one of their features, deception. We mean, therefore, to claim for deception, lying, and dissemblance no more than its due as part of the "natural" feature of our environment. Our task is not to decide whether deception should or should not exist, but rather to understand the nature and function of deception in our intra- and interpersonal lives.

Elsewhere, distinctions between kinds of deception have been offered; for example, deception that serves to protect the self from punishment, or deception to spare the feelings of another. Deception to spare the feelings of another can range all the way from the false lover's claim that his infidelity, if exposed, will hurt his girlfriend's feelings, to the young child who says to her arthritic grandmother that she enjoyed the sweater that the grandmother knitted even when she did not. While we believe the deception of the little girl in lying about her grandmother's sweater is based on saving the feelings of another, we are somewhat troubled by the claims of the boyfriend. Is his deception designed to avoid punishment for himself, the anger and upset of his girlfriend, or is it truly the case that his deception is designed to avoid hurting his girlfriend's feelings? Is his deception based on an awareness of giving pain to his girlfriend or is it based on his self-deception, that is, his unaware motive to avoid pain or punishment?

While many different taxonomies about deception can be offered, we have chosen the following division, based on a consideration of the state of the deceiver's awareness of their deception as well as the subject of the deceiver's action. For the sake of discussion about lying in everyday experience, we have chosen to distinguish between three types of deception: (1) ordinary deception toward others committed with self-awareness; (2) deception toward others that requires some degree of self-deception; and (3) self-deception even in the absence of another, that is, the need for illusion. It is clear that many taxonomies, other than the ones we have provided, could be built around the topic of deception. Notice that in this taxonomy, we distinguish between deception *toward* another and deception *toward* ourselves and aware versus unaware deception. These two dimensions create the taxonomy that we present here. This taxonomy will be useful in understanding the chapters that make up this volume.

Deception with Self-Awareness

Examples of deception directed toward others are common. Children tell their parents that they have done their chores even though they have not, so as to avoid the anger and punishment of their parents. Students tell their teachers that a friend was sick so they could not finish their assignment on time. Couples living together often tell each other things that they know not to be true.

In most of these examples, deception of this type is designed to avoid anger of or punishment by others for not doing what we know we should do (or should not do). The deceiver knows what was expected of him/her and seeks to hide the failure to meet the expectations from the other. The deceiver also knows what is in the mind of the other; thus the deception is specifically designed to fool or hide his/her actions from the other. It is such types of deception that more often than not are subject to societal scorn. Such phrases as, "You ought to be brave enough to take your punishment if you didn't do what you should or if you did something you shouldn't," is the familiar form of our feeling about such types of deception.

We are offended at the deception for two reasons: first, the reason itself for the deception, namely, the failure of the individual to act (or not act) in such a way so as to fulfill the obligation, duty, or expected action. This failure could be a moral failure or it could simply be a failure of obligation. The second reason for the scorn associated with such deception is that it reflects on the interpersonal relationship. Such an idea is captured by the phrase, "You lied to me." Here we see that the focus of the scorn is not so much the failure of the particular action, thought, or desire, but the interpersonal failure associated with lying to the other. We believe that people in significant relationships—friends, parents and children, husbands and wives, lovers—should not lie to one another; lying destroys the fabric and trust of the relationship. This type of deception is used as an example of the destructive nature of lying and deception since it reflects interpersonal failure (see Bok, 1978, for example). Although such deception is quite common and may well be built into the fabric of our psychic lives, it is understandable how we become quite upset over the lies or deception of another. The loss of interpersonal trust associated with the lie seems to be the important focal point.

While we cannot sympathize with such types of deception, they are readily understandable. Consider that there may be some adaptive significance in avoiding punishment and harm even for one's transgression. If this were true, then lying becomes a natural consequence of the failure that leads to the lie. The adaptive significance of lying can be seen in the following example. If you lived in a society that believed that punishment for stealing should be the cutting off of your hand, you would not likely confess to stealing, especially if your action had been unobserved. You would in all probability lie in order to avoid such horrible punishment. In some sense the lie is adaptive. For this reason, it is important to make a distinction between the act of lying and the transgression that led to the lie. While it is wrong for individuals to steal and may not be adaptive for them to do so, it is adaptive for them to lie about it, if it helps avoid punishment.

The distinction between the transgression that led to the lie and the lie itself is often not made when the lie involves two people.

Parents are often quite upset when their children lie. In part, this is because they focus on the the act of lying as reflecting interpersonal failure rather than on the transgression itself. Occasionally one hears parents saying, "But she lied to me." It matters little that lying may be an adaptive response that children use or that the child is normal. By focusing on the interpersonal relationship the lie endangers, we often fail to consider the transgression itself.

Little Susie who steals Gellie's doll and lies about it has committed two transgressions—stealing the toy and lying about it to her mother. It seems reasonable that our attention should be drawn to the transgression, for if there were no transgression, there would be no lie. Susie needs to be taught not to steal. This lesson is often lost in the anger over the lie. Ron lies to Jan about his affair. While we consider his infidelity and lie shameful, we can readily understand it. We lie to protect ourselves. Our moral sense requires that we not lie; however, few of us are saints.

Deception Toward Others That Requires Self-Deception

We can deceive others and not be aware that we are doing so. This kind of deception can include deceiving others about ourselves, deceiving others about others, and deceptions about others to others, all of which we are not aware. The important feature in these kinds of deceptions is our lack of awareness about the deception, which raises a troublesome question. How can there be unaware deception? For deception to take place the deceiver has to know that something is true and at the same time act as if it is not true. By definition it would appear that unaware deception is impossible. The issue of aware versus unaware deception when translated into the language of conscious versus unconscious awareness allows us to escape this difficulty. Since Freud, our commitment to these two different types of awareness, both of them existing within our own psyche, provides the means by which we can examine classes of deception of which we are unaware.

Unaware deception exists at many levels. At the most extreme end of our psyche is the phenomenon of multiple personality disorders. People who suffer from this disorder are capable of deceiving themselves as well as others and this deceiving of others can take place over entire lifetimes. On a more common everyday level, we may deceive others and simply not be aware of our own deception. For example, one can compliment another on that person's looks or what that person said and not mean it, but be unaware of it. Or consider the husband who deceives his wife about an extramarital affair and does so because he feels that to tell her would hurt her feelings. In some sense he knows he is deceiving his wife, yet he deceives himself into thinking that the reason why he is deceiving her is for her own good; in fact, it is for his good. The psychic battle between conscious and unconscious awareness makes itself felt in these kinds of distinction. Many examples of this type of deception are possible and parallel closely those that have awareness. The major difference between this and the first class of deception is in the person's recognition and awareness that he/she is intentionally deceiving another.

Self-Deception

The idea of self-deception poses the same difficulty as does unaware deception toward others. The question, "How can it be that the self can deceive itself," remains with us. The answer, as we have already seen, rests in postulating different aspects or features of the self. Freud's tripartite psyche, in which different aspects of the self can be in conflict, allows us to consider self-deception. The topic of self-deception rests on a psychic division in which some features are aware while others are not. The process of self-deception, like other processes such as denial, repression, or reaction formation, and many more, rests on this same feature. Unless we are prepared to postulate that there is one aspect of the self that can deny or repress information to another aspect of the self, we will be unable to accept the idea of self-deception.

We can deceive ourselves for a variety of reasons, one of the most important of which is to avoid the lowering of our self-esteem or to avoid shame. For example, take the young man who calls a young woman up for a date, and is told that she is busy for the next three weekends. He now has a choice of how to interpret that information. He can conclude that she does not want to go out with him, and feel humiliated, embarrassed, or shamed. Alternatively, he can conclude that such a busy person is not convenient to date and, therefore, he does not want to date her. This spares him the psychic pain of shame or humiliation. It seems clear that the major reasons for self-deception have to do with avoiding negative feelings about the self.

The psychic advantage of this attitude seems clear. For certain circumstances there may be little reason to lower one's self-esteem by "being honest with the one's self." In such circumstances, the psychic cost of shame, humiliation, or embarrassment may be greater than the psychic advantage in not deceiving the self. For example, if you were at a restaurant and committed some breach of etiquette but learned how to behave in the future, it might be of psychic advantage to play down the significance of the mistake, especially since you would have already learned from the experience and since thinking about the mistake would result in further humiliation.

On the other hand, self-deception can be very costly for the individual, for the very reason that the deception may prevent you from learning from or rectifying your mistake. For example, suppose in examining your body you discover a lump and decide that the lump had always been present. Under such a strategy no action would likely be taken. But should the lump be an indication of the beginning of breast cancer, such self-deception could result in serious consequences and even death.

There are reasons to assume that self-deception can be advantageous as well as disadvantageous, and only a careful analysis of self-deception can disentangle the problem. However, there is no question that self-deception—the creation of illusions, "looking at the world through rose-colored spectacles"—has its advantage. Because of this, we cannot readily accept the idea that all forms of self-deception or other similar psychic phenomena like denial or forgetting are necessarily maladaptive.

MORAL ISSUES IN DECEPTION

The word "lying," especially in this country, has a very powerful negative connotation. If you call someone a liar, you deliver a very significant insult. Given that so many people, in so many circumstances, are prone to lie, it is rather strange that this term is so offensive. Whether or not the aversion to lying is a universal characteristic, and we believe it is, to some degree, in the United States lying is considered a very significant negative activity. To gain some idea of the American attitude, think about the myth concerning the founding father, liberating general, and first President of the United States, George Washington. All school children learn it; it is the single most known fact about George Washington's early childhood: he did not tell a lie. As the story goes, George Washington, when he was a young man, took an axe and chopped down a cherry tree. When his father asked him about it, George said something to the effect, "I cannot tell a lie, I chopped down the cherry tree." Since every child is told he could be president, Washington's truth-telling remains fixed in the mind as prerequisite for the task. That this is the best known story of Washington's early childhood reflects, in part, on the American concern with this question of lying and with the strong negative connotation associated with it. In attempt to avoid using the

word "lie," we often substitute such terms as "deception," "dissembling," or "masking."

This book is not concerned with the moral issues regarding lying
or deception. It can be easily argued that lying is an immoral act;
indeed many people believe it is. That there are different types or
degrees of deception is still for some people irrelevant to the question
of morality; lying in order to spare the feelings of another is still a lie.
For others, lying to spare the feelings of another constitutes a higher
form of moral behavior than does the simple injunction to always tell
the truth. It is beyond the purview of this book to settle such
differences. What we can do is to point out different types of lying, the
behaviors associated with them, the outcomes, and the circumstances
in which they occur.

Because there has been no careful study of changes in societal
behaviors related to lying and deception, we have to rely on more
casual observation in order to determine if there have been any
historical or cultural changes in our attitudes to lying. One place to
look is the subject of etiquette, which reveals that one of the very
important consequences of "behaving properly" is that it allows us to
act quite independently of how we feel or think. Thus, for example, as
a guest in someone's house for dinner, it is appropriate etiquette to
thank the host for the lovely meal even though it might not have been
an enjoyable one. Prescribed and predetermined behavior allows us to
act in ways that are not congruent with the way we think or feel; as
such, etiquette can be considered to be a form of deception.

The importance of behaving properly, independently of how we
wish to behave, has a long history in this country; books of etiquette
were transported from the Old World. What is of interest is the current
status of etiquette. The 1960s in the United States stressed personal
freedom and respect for the individual, and the idea that etiquette was
inappropriate since it was often in the service of deceptive behavior.
The ethos of that time required that we should not deceive one
another, even for the sake of sparing the other's feelings. Because of
this, fewer books on etiquette were read and written and emphasis on
appropriate behavior, independently of how we really thought or felt,
was discouraged. If an individual was honest and true to his or her
beliefs and feelings, then, regardless of what those beliefs and feelings
were, they deserved to be expressed, and the cost of such behavior was
something that needed to be borne by the individual involved. (It
should be noticed that this concept now has lost some of its moral and
psychological certainty.) The importance of etiquette has once more
become popular, as witnessed by the increased popularity of such
books. The point to be made is that cultural values, such as etiquette,

show us that the American displeasure with the lie, while presently high, changes with the mood of the times.

We have been stressing American culture when discussing lying. But lying and deception are universal human characteristics and it is evident that all cultures employ deception and lying to some extent. For example, in the United States we believe in emotional expressivity; that is, we believe that to express feelings is a positive and virtuous act. We are quite willing to act emotionally to one another as well as to ourselves. However, we know that other cultures are much less apt to act emotionally. For example, the Japanese do not believe that emotional expressivity is a positive act and so they mask their emotions, and thus they behave in a way different from how they may feel.

The expression of anger is an example of cultural diversity in the expression of emotion. In the United States, the expression of anger, although considered at times inappropriate, is tolerated. In Japan, however, the expression of anger is unacceptable. Japanese withhold their angry emotion. Is it fair then to say that those Japanese who do not express their anger, even though they are angry, are using deception? To an American, such deception might seem pathological. An American might be urged by his friends to seek therapy so that he could learn to let others know about his feelings or to learn the truth about himself; that is, his lack of expression of anger demonstrates that he is deceiving himself.

We can think of many other cultural differences in the use of lying and deception. One particular example comes readily to mind, having to do with how different cultures engage in commercial activities such as the buying and selling of goods. In the United States, for the most part, the price on an object is the price that the consumer must pay. Even here, however, we recognize that the price shown may be deceptive. How much more true is this in cultures in which bargaining is the rule. For example, when the seller says, "This is my final price," is she not lying in the same way as when the purchaser says, "This is my final price," and starts to walk away? The entire bargaining process is a series of deceptions, ritualized into a technique in which goods are bought and sold.

Such examples as these indicate that there are different cultural rules pertaining to lying and deception, the existence of which does not speak to different moral senses but rather to the basic premises that underlie human behavior. One cannot help marvelling at the extent of lying and deception that humans engage in, especially when we consider the various techniques that humans have evolved for successful social exchanges. One of us (Lewis) is reminded of something his grandmother told him many years ago. Her advice was to deceive in a very special way, in order to maintain friendships. When asked how your vacation was, she advised the best answer you could give would be to say that it had been terrible, even if it had not. By saying it was terrible, rather than enjoyable, you were more likely to avoid the jealousy of your friends and more likely to elicit sympathetic responses. It was her belief that bragging or even telling the truth, especially if something very good had occurred, endangered social relationships. Whether or not such grandmotherly advice should be valued is debatable. What it does point out, however, is the complexity of human interactions and the role that deception and lying may play.

VARIATIONS WITHIN LYING AND DECEPTION

So far we have addressed lying, deception, and illusions in terms of rather general patterns. It is obvious that people differ in how they deceive, lie, or maintain illusions. As psychologists, we are interested in looking at subpatterns within the larger patterns, and these subpatterns often reflect traditional cultural categories, such as age, group, and gender, but they can also be constructed around interesting categories such as "who has control" or "who has the most to lose." Subpatterns in deception also occur relative to the general division between that which is adaptive and that which is maladaptive (although this judgment of degree of adaptiveness may well depend on the perspectives of the people involved, namely, whether one is the deceiver or the target of the deception). We will briefly describe some of these subpatterns or "who does what" in deception, but the reader would do well to read the other contributions in this volume to get a fuller grasp of some of the fascinating subpatterns to be found in lying and deception.

Age Differences in Deception

We will not address age differences in *detection* of deception here, rather we are interested in how age can be used as a general indicator of onset of different types of deception. For example, symbolic pretend play emerges in the early preschool years and can be thought of as a type of illusion. Imaginary friends may be used as illusory culprits when one's three-year-old is questioned about how lipstick got smeared all over the bathroom sink.

Lying to Avoid Punishment. One of us (Lewis) details in Chapter 4 how lying to avoid punishment in an experimental situation can be observed to occur in children as young as two years of age. By the time a child is four years of age, lying to avoid possible punishment is a readily undertaken strategy.

Cheating in School. This type of deception is not designed to avoid punishment but rather to gain advantages for oneself without having to expend the effort otherwise needed to acquire those advantages legitimately, and it is readily apparent in the earliest grades. Cheating by children in the early elementary school years may be somewhat easier to detect (e.g., when they have rather obviously copied somebody else's work), but the older child is able to take into account the "informational needs" of the observer (e.g., the teacher) and thus can more readily avoid detection.

Emotional Dissemblance. Putting on an emotional front, a form of emotional–expressive deception which one of us (Saarni) has elaborated in another chapter, also appears to have its precursors in about the third year, as when one's preschooler exaggerates his pain from a trivial injury in order to get parental attention. By middle childhood, children can competently talk about how one must hide one's fear when faced by a bully or simulate pleasure when one's grandparent has given one socks again for one's birthday. They can readily take into account who will be made vulnerable if one's real emotions are expressed: oneself or one's interactant (as in hurting someone's feelings by revealing one's own real feelings). Interestingly, children are most likely to refer to intensity of emotion as the prime reason for genuinely expressing feelings, in spite of social sanctions or social risks, due to the sense of uncontrollability of the intense emotion.

Self-Deception. Self-deception in childhood has received little empirical research attention, although the literature based on adults is considerably richer (for example, see Baumeister's and Solomon's chapters in this volume). Adolescents are clearly capable of it, but exactly how self-deception manifests itself in early-to-middle child-hood is less obvious. Clinical evidence suggests that the kinds of defense mechanisms commonly used by children (e.g., repression, denial, and regression) may also function as self-deceptive strategies. For example, the seven-year-old, who knows full well that once something is dead it does not come back to life, may be terrified of burying her dead hamster for fear it will "suffocate" under the earth. As with adults, self-deception often aids wishful thinking and may manifest itself as denial of the obvious. However, self-deception in children may also have the function of facilitating children's ability to cope with very painful and distressing circumstances or to avoid shame and humiliation. It is common, for example, for children whose parents are going through a divorce to deny that anything is "wrong" with their family, or they may maintain that Daddy has only gone away on a trip, despite both parents' attempts at clear communication to the contrary.

Manipulation. Children's manipulative strategies to control other people's behavior toward them are also variations on the theme of deception. For example, one of us (Saarni) worked therapeutically with a five-year-old client to help the child deal more adaptively with her ostensible separation anxiety from her mother. Prior to her mother's recent remarriage, Suzanna [not her real name] often had the privilege of sleeping with Mom. Now, since that was no longer an option for her, she developed terrifying nightmares of huge hands coming out from the cracks of her closet door dripping with blood and, of course, they were coming right for her. Her response was to go screaming out into the hall, get down on the floor in front of the couple's bedroom door, and get her mouth lined up with the crack under the door. Then she would begin a two-hour litany of how much she loved and missed her mother, how scared she was, how bad her mother was for not taking care of her, and so forth (omitting the stepfather from all her laments).

The mother had already tried a number of reasonable interventions before scheduling her daughter's counseling appointment. During the very first session with Suzanna, while working together with crayons, paints, and clay, Suzanna revealed that she made up the dreams just as she was able to make up scary pictures to paint or draw. At that point, pragmatism and concern for the parents' nonexistent medical insurance benefits led to the following successful intervention: a small pet that could sleep in Suzanna's room was recommended. She acquired almost immediately a little rabbit and the ostensible nightmares and crying outside in the hall stopped that very same night and did not resume because, in Suzanna's words, "I didn't want to wake up Bunny." Thus, once the advantages to be gained (or disadvantages to be avoided) are no longer relevant or have been replaced by a gratifying substitute, a specific deceptive manipulative strategy should subside in children's behavior.

Excuse-making. Learning to make excuses, a common type of "white lie" in our culture (see Sigmon and Snyder, Chapter 7, this volume), has also been infrequently investigated in childhood. The most noteworthy research was undertaken by Weiner and Handel (1985), who determined that children were most likely to give excuses related to *uncontrollable* events as the reasons why they had to break a scheduled play date (which for children is tantamount to social rejection). Thus, getting sick or blaming one's mother for being unable to get together with another child were typical uncontrollable events cited by school-age children, as opposed to saying that they preferred to do something else or had lost interest in playing with the peer.

The general conclusion to be drawn about subpatterns created in deception by the influence of age group is that it seems to be primarily a degree of strategic finesse. Young children can lie; they can emotionally mask their feelings and manipulate, give excuses, create illusions for themselves, and even deceive themselves. The fact that quite young children are capable of lying to avoid punishment suggests that the capacity for deception is probably pan-cultural, a topic to which we will return below.

Social Roles: The Influence of Gender

The contribution by DePaulo, Epstein, and Wyer to this volume (Chapter 6) represents "the state of the art" when it comes to summarizing some of the typical sex differences found in deception in our culture. The pattern they describe most generally characterizes the lies committed by women as focusing on the feelings of others, putting a "positive gloss" on events, or falsely derogating oneself so as to prop up the ego of the other. Men's lies are more self-centered and sometimes they even pretend to be more disgruntled or gruff than they feel in order to maneuver people into acting the way they want them to.

Women also tend to be more likely "not to see" the lies communicated by others; it is as though they would rather not stir things up (in themselves or within the relationship) by detecting the lie; thus the possibility of being more self-deceptive may exist. Men are more likely to confront the deception, or, at the very least, pay attention to giveaway clues and entertain the suspicion that the other is attempting to deceive them.

The effect of gender on lying is also evident in research undertaken by the British sociologist, Annette Lawson, who examined sex differences in adultery and especially in the matter of who tells whom about the adulterous events (Lawson, 1988). She examined the interpersonal dynamics of deception by looking at how spouses either reveal or conceal their extramarital sexual activities, as captured by the following trenchant quote from one of her research participants:

> I made him swear he'd always tell me nothing but the truth. I promised him I never would resent it. No matter how unbearable, how harsh, how cruel. How come he thought I meant it? (p. 224)

The woman quoted above is incredulous that her husband, in reality, would not lie to her to protect her feelings or put a positive gloss on his infidelity. But the quote is also noteworthy for indicating, as Lawson goes on to document, that in recent years it is more often husbands who "confess" their extramarital sex than wives. Lawson makes a simple and reasonable argument as to why men tell and women do not, and her survey subjects essentially say the same thing: Women have a lot more to lose if they tell than men do. Cultural history has supported this differential power, with women in not so distant times even being legally killed by their husbands if they were found to be adulterous, and husbands often being excused for their sexual infidelities.

Interestingly, Lawson also found sex differences in the nature of the extramarital affair when confessions to the spouse were made. Men were not so likely to tell about their one-night stands or other short-term (less than six months) affairs and were more likely to reveal their more significant and longer-lasting extramarital relationships; in other words, those that would appear to threaten the marital bond most in terms of intimacy and, on some level, commitment to the lover. On the other hand, women were not likely to reveal their significant long-term relationships. But their deception of their spouse bothered them, whereas husbands were less bothered by their deception. Women's resolution to their discomfort with deception tended to be either to end the affair or the marriage. From DePaulo and associates' essay (Chapter 6) and from Lawson's work on adultery, the pattern we seem to discern most clearly in women's deception is a focus on the emotion at hand, whether it is protecting the feelings of another or her own emotional investment. Men's deception seems more task-oriented, more concretely functional. This is not to say that women necessarily feel more ashamed over deception than men do, rather we suspect that the emotional consequences of deception vary for men and women, depending on the interpersonal connection involved and depending on whether guilt or shame is involved. Surprisingly, there has been relatively little empirical research into what these gender-based differences in emotion sequelae to deception are, although Lewis (1992), in discussing shame, has suggested one. Women more than men are likely to blame themselves over a transgression. A woman would be more likely to say, "I lied, I'm no good," but a man would be more likely to say, "I didn't lie, it was partially true" or "I lied but you made me do it." In either case, women, more than men, would blame themselves. Moreover, women are likely to make an evaluation about their total selves while men make an evaluation about their actions. Because of this, women are more likely to feel shame ("I'm no good") while men are likely to feel guilt or regret ("What I did was no good").

Deception in Non-Western Cultures

We wanted to describe some instances of deception in several non-Western cultures, which are also not industrialized, as a way of emphasizing once again the ubiquity of deception in human experience. In our discussions of this topic with anthropologists Sue Parker and Tom Rosin (1992), what emerged was that in simple societies when deception occurs, it is typically around aggression or dominance, access to food or goods, access to desirable mates, or, interestingly, between men and women around what we might call "gender knowledge" (e.g., women may conceal from men or deny knowing how to use contraceptive strategies while men may conceal from women knowledge about hunting strategies or some religious rituals). They also noted that anthropologists have themselves been at times deliberately misinformed by their informants, perhaps accounting for some of the widely discrepant descriptions of some cultural practices; for example, Passin (1942) determined that his informant lied to him about sorcery practices and whipping of children.

To illustrate deception in aggressive or dominance contexts, Eibl-Eibesfeldt (1971) describes the Waika Indians of the Upper Orinoco holding mock battles when the inhabitants of one village visit another. This mock battle was used between friendly villages as a way to defuse potential conflict and threat and thus avoid serious injury and damage. Taking one's family into the village was another way of showing one's friendly intent, but on occasion this was a ruse, and the village was attacked anyway.

Deception around one's goods, food, and even children can be seen in how cultures deal with envy. Envy in a peasant culture has been examined by Foster (1972), who theorized that in cultures with an implicit or explicit "economic" view that there was only a limited quantity of goods to be distributed, the experience of envy in oneself would be controlled, suppressed, or denied, and one would attempt to safeguard oneself against another's envy, whether it was directed at one's material goods or at one's advantage in having children. The "evil eye," which is symbolic for envy in several cultures, was avoided by hiding one's desirable material goods from onlookers who might come to covet them; or, according to an account of the Aritama in Colombia: "The best prophylactic measure an individual can take . . . consists in not appearing enviable in the first place and in pretending to be poor, ill, and already in trouble" (Foster, 1972, p. 175). Foster also makes an interesting analysis of why compliments may make us uncomfortable: they may make us aware of others' envy of and resentful feelings toward our good fortune. Their envy of us brings with it the risk that they might try to undermine or acquire our good fortune for themselves. Hence, it is common in many diverse cultures when receiving a compliment to deny the basis of the compliment or belittle its validity.

Suppression or denial of envy toward another in the peasant cultures studied by Foster typically took the form of denouncing bad luck, fate, or assorted deities and witches for one's own inferior situation rather than admitting to feeling envy at another's well-being and thereby confronting one's subordinate status and humiliation. As Foster points out, it is a lot more bearable to say that one has been dealt a "bad blow" by fate (or that some spirits have it in for you), rather than to acknowledge that one's deprivation or disadvantage is a result of one's own shortcomings (p. 184).

Access to desirable mates has a long history of deceptive ploys and ruses. For example, Chagnon (1983) describes the chieftains of the rain forest Yanomano Indians (Venezuela and Brazil) as manipulating the kinship rules about whom one was permitted to marry by "redefining" kinship relations to their own advantage, thus permitting marriages to be arranged that otherwise would have been classified as incestuous and therefore prohibited. Yanomano infidelities were carried out as follows: "Clandestine sexual liaisons usually take place at this time of day [early morning], having been arranged on the previous evening. The lovers leave the village on the pretext of 'going to the toilet' and meet at some predetermined location. They return to the village by opposite routes" (p. 117).

Concealment of certain kinds of knowledge from the opposite sex has been found among several cultures; sometimes the concealment is based on the notion that something is taboo (e.g., to reveal the knowledge would bring bad luck or bad spirits), but more frequently it occurs as sex-segregated rituals, such as boys' initiation rites, men's hunting ceremonies, birthing, and menstruation. Marjorie Shostak's (1981) interviews with the !Kung woman, Nisa, indicated that among the bushmen, boys were isolated from women for several weeks while they prepared for "Choma," the male initiation rite, during which "ritual knowledge of male matters is passed from one generation to the next" (p. 239). Women were also prohibited from handling certain kinds of equipment, especially if they were also menstruating, and most bushmen healers were also men.

Ellen Basso's extensive observations of the Brazilian Indian group, the Kalapalo, also indicated that men concealed certain kinds of knowledge and ritual from women, who, in turn, concealed birthing practices from men (Basso, 1973, 1987). She describes in some detail the *kagutu* or trumpet-blowing ceremony "played by men and forbidden to the sight of women on pain of mass rape" (1973, p. 60) and suggests that its primary function was as a ritual marker of male differentiation from females.

The above examples of "knowledge" that one gender conceals from the other do not sound at all similar to what men and women might systematically conceal from one another in our culture, but, upon closer examination, we can think of contemporary examples that suggest similar gender-based deceptive strategies. Perhaps one of the most obvious is clubs that permit male members only. In recent years, many exclusive men's clubs have begun to admit women members, as women have applied pressure on them to open up access to one of the "benefits" that often comes with such club membership, namely, inside information about business strategies, opportunities for persuasive maneuvers, financial advantages, and so forth.

Lastly, feigning an emotion that is not really felt is a deceptive practice found in virtually all cultures. Sometimes the contradiction between the expressive display and the subjective feeling is explained as being caused by ghosts or spirits, but often it is acknowledged simply as what is proper, especially when the expressive display is directed at a higher ranking individual. For example, Samoans, Balinese, and Tahitians have all been described as having private and public selves, although their definition of self is much more fluid than ours and is more likely to be defined by the relationships they have with others. Their public presentation has been described as emotionally composed, but privately they admitted to concerns with somatic disturbance and internal feelings were acknowledged (Levy, 1973).

On the one hand, there appears to be considerable variety in deceptive behavior across both Western and non-Western cultures; on the other hand, there appear to be some common patterns as well. Deceit around clandestine affairs, protection of one's "turf" by misleading one's competitor, and feigning an emotion that one does not feel seem to be the most frequently encountered kinds of deception. However, our generalization needs to be tempered with the qualification that, to our knowledge, a meta-analysis of cross-cultural data involving deception has not been undertaken. However, as Mitchell shows us (in Chapter 3), even some nonhuman primates can lie, and certainly there are many other animals that have been endowed with camouflaging coloration or the ability to mislead predators. Thus, misleading appearances and deception in general can very likely be found in all societies.

When Lying Hurts the Liar

We will address two kinds of maladaptive deception here: malingering and excessive emotional dissemblance. The first topic is extensively addressed by Kropp and Rogers in this volume (Chapter 10), and the latter is further examined by Saarni and von Salisch in their contribution (Chapter 5).

Malingering. At one time or another, most of us have pretended to be sick, overtired, or too depressed in order to avoid obligations. We expect that most readers have also experienced the following: A situation becomes much more emotionally manageable if one can avoid it or postpone dealing with it until one feels more adequate. We do not think such occasional lapses are particularly maladaptive; in fact, they may even provide much needed respite, as when a social worker calls in sick but readily discloses she needs the day off for the sake of her sanity. The kind of malingering that does become maladaptive is when it is chronic and essentially develops into a lifestyle of avoidance or when it is frequently used as a lie to cover for one's responsibility in assorted misdeeds.

The malingering person living an avoidant lifestyle is in a precarious position: He or she must maintain the posture of the sick person to others, regardless of how close a relationship they might have, and seek confirmation from "experts" as a way to justify the avoidance to the self as well as to others. To let down the pretense, even for a moment, is to invite shame and humiliation—a rather dire emotional state that most of us dread.

What is it that the malingerer seeks to avoid? Kropp and Rogers (Chapter 10, this volume), suggest a model with three features that characterize the malingering person's "beliefs": (1) He or she believes that some anticipated event, which centrally involves the self, is threatening and adversarial; (2) he or she believes that a truthful disclosure will be disadvantageous to the self; and (3) he or she does not believe that alternative means exist for reaching the desired goal of protecting the self. Thus, what successful malingerers avoid is risk to the self but, in so doing, they also lose the benefits that may go along with some degree of risk to the self (e.g., feelings of competence and high self-esteem upon accomplishing a difficult and challenging task). But malingerers have to deal with anxiety about exposure of their feigned illness or disability, and so while malingering is used to avoid anxiety-provoking risk to the self, its use brings with it inherent anxiety about the possibility of discovery and subsequent shame.

The kind of malingering used to avoid responsibility and blame for harm to others is found typically in criminal cases or in the reports of child protective services. Kropp and Rogers describe the careful and planned simulation of multiple personalities by the Hillside Strangler as a ruse developed by him to avoid criminal conviction. More recently, a serial murderer of young men in the Midwest announced his plea of insanity as part of the ongoing trial. Given the sensational nature of the admissions by these grotesquely horrible serial murderers, chronic malingering to avoid responsibility for one's misdeeds might seem relatively rare, but given the variety of circumstances where this occurs, we suggest it is more common than at first thought.

The claim that "I can't remember because I drank too much" has been a common thread in many physical and sexual abuse reports: alcohol is "blamed" for the perpetrator's acts and is the reason why the perpetrator believes himself to be blameless in abusing his child. It was not his "real" self that harmed the child. Substance abuse does indeed impair judgement, but it also contributes to a variation on the theme of malingering in that the substance-abusing person believes him- or herself to be facing an adversarial event (e.g., an evaluation by a child protective service social worker), that he has something to lose if he is truthful, and that he does not perceive an alternative way of avoiding blame for a misdeed.

Maladaptive Emotional Dissemblance. Rigid, inflexible, and chronic "emotional fronts" create problems for the person using them. Chief among these problems is that the sorts of relationships the person has with others are rarely anxiety-free or satisfying. Individuals who adopt an emotional mask that is virtually never taken off experience considerable isolation and trepidation over their impostor selves. Like the malingerer, the threat of exposure is high and the dread of shame is ever-present (see also Lewis, 1992).

Consider the following case: Diane [not her real name] was a police officer in a department that was predominantly male and mostly white; Diane was bicultural (African-American and European). Beginning with her training and extending through her advancement to officer status, Diane always felt she had to present herself to her fellow officers as tougher, more cynical, and more "unflappable" than they were and certainly more so than she felt on the inside. The result after some six years of police work was a social exterior that was abrasive, distancing, and decidedly unsympathetic. However, on the inside, revealed during her counseling sessions, Diane felt terribly and painfully lonely, perceived herself as walking on eggshells around her co-workers lest they discover how vulnerable she really felt; her self-esteem was readily shaken by the slightest hint of criticism, and she suffered frequent somatic maladies, some rather serious. Even when not at work, Diane either had to maintain her emotional front with other off-duty officers or literally be alone. Increasingly she chose the latter, becoming more depressed and also drinking more. Finally, despair led her to quit police work, and she moved to another state as well.

The point to make here relative to the maladaptiveness of excessive and inflexible emotional masking is that it can contribute to tremendous internal emotional distress. It can also create misleading assumptions on the part of others about the individual who maintains such a rigid emotional front. Stoicism as an emotional front may have a role in some situations, but its application across the board and without taking into account the specifics of interpersonal relationships can lead to increased rather than diminished anguish.

Maladaptive forms of deception have been looked at here from the standpoint of what lying does to the deceiver, especially with regard to how splitting of the self into inside/outside selves or real versus imposter selves contributes to anxiety over exposure and resulting shame. This is not to minimize in any way the pain and loss to many victims of deception and lies. We have also not considered here the loss of trust when the deceiver is found out by her or his intended targets of deceit. The deceiver is then likely to be rejected and/or punished, and the quality of relationship between deceiver and deceived typically deteriorates. "Lies that fail" are described in detail by Ekman and Frank (Chapter 9), and they elaborate the contexts and cues which accompany lies that can be detected or that are unsuccessful.

THE LYING SELF

Up to this point, much of what we have said about lying has emphasized the social significance of lying. Except for self-deception, most other forms of lying and deception, including masking our feelings, are designed to affect our social relationships. While this is certainly the case, it is also important to note that the act of lying or deception involves elaborate cognitive ability. Consider deception in the service of avoiding punishment. A student enters her professor's office. The professor is sitting at her desk and has the student's term paper in front of her. She asks the student to be seated and says "Linda, did you write this paper by yourself?" We know that Linda has had help. Linda looks at the teacher and says "Yes, I did write it myself." In order for Linda to be successful in her deception, she must carry out several cognitive activities and do so successfully in order to avoid punishment.

First, she must deny that she has cheated on the paper. While this appears obvious at first, it is something that has to be learned. For example, very young children under the age of four when asked if they have done something wrong are more apt to admit it than when they get older. We have to learn not to admit to something that we should not do so as not to get into trouble. While such learning is very simple and takes place quickly, nonetheless it requires that we learn this rule.

Second, Linda must manage her appearance, in terms of facial expression and vocal behavior, as well as body posture. Linda has to act as if she is telling the truth. This means that Linda has to know what an "innocent" appearance looks like. From the point of view of the cultural norms she must adapt her appearance to conform with known rules. The masking or altering of one's appearance including voice, face, and body are skills which also are acquired early. For example, in Chapter 4, Lewis shows that children as young as three years of age are quite successful in masking their emotional expressions, so much so that observers have a difficult time in detecting their lying.

Thirdly, in order to be successful in her lie, Linda has to know something about what the professor knows in regard to Linda's behavior. (E.g., the professor might have other samples of Linda's writing skills or performance on exams; Linda may need to come up with plausible explanations for why her term paper surpasses the quality of her previously submitted work.) This requires that Linda be able to think about what it is that is in the mind of another. This ability to think about one's self and to think about other selves standing alone or in relationship to ourselves is an important cognitive capacity which appears to emerge somewhere around the third year of life.

Because lying taps into these elaborate cognitive capacities, the study of and interest in lying does not rest solely on its social significance. Children's ability to lie informs us about what they know about the rules, especially those they have violated, and what they know others know about the rules or about deceptive behavior. It is no wonder then, for those people interested in studying the process of thinking or interested in how children acquire theories of mind, that the study of lying is a significant tool with which to explore these questions.

One important cognitive feature that emerges from the study of lying is the concept of self. Being able to lie or deceive implies intention. Whether conscious or unconscious or aware or unaware, deception is an active process whereby the deceiver *intends* to deceive. Although other forms of deception, such as camouflage, do not involve intention in the form we usually think of it, deception in humans does. Because deception and lying involve intention, the study of deception also informs us about the nature of selves. An intentional act implies that a person has what we commonly call objective self-awareness; that is, the organism has the capacity to reflect on its own behavior. In deception, the person not only reflects on his/her own behavior but reflects upon how that behavior will affect another's behavior. In other words, lying and deception imply a self-referential system. Self-referential systems develop (Lewis, 1992; Lewis & Michalson, 1983). We would expect, from an ontogenic perspective, that children should be unable to intentionally deceive until after the second year of life. From a phylogenetic point of view, organisms should not show intentionally deceptive behavior unless they have a self-referential system. Given our information about the great apes—that orangutans, gorillas, and chimpanzees have a self-reflecting system—it is not surprising that there is evidence that indicates deception in these creatures.

It is important, however, to make clear that there are different levels of deception. As Mitchell (Chapter 3) and Solomon (Chapter 2) put it, the cognitive capacities vary as a function of the type of deception seen. None of us would accept the deceptive behavior of an insect's change of coloring as the same kind of deception as Linda's in denying she cheated on her term paper. In the same way, we argue that there are different levels of cognitive capacity which underlie these behaviors. In particular, we look for differences in the self-systems of these organisms.

Finally, deception and lying bear upon the issue of the nature of minds. We have already noticed that in order for self-deception to take place, we need to postulate a type of mind which has, by its nature, compartments. In other words, the model of mind that appears to best fit the data of our experience is an un-unified set of distinct parts. The idea of the self as a unity, a singular thing in opposition to other such singular things, is a uniquely Western view (Geertz, 1984).

Perhaps no more dramatic an example of the multiple aspects of ourselves can be found than in the clinical work surrounding multiple personality disorders. Assuming the phenomenon is real, what we see in this phenomenon is the possibility that multiple "people" with different motives, desires, and needs can all be housed in the same person. Even more remarkably, some of these different people are aware of others but are not all aware of each other. Such a phenomenon alerts us to the need to develop a model about selves which utilizes the information both from our clinical experiences as well as from phenomena such as self-deception.

In the following chapters, some of the leading investigators of the phenomena of lying and deception present their particular views. While it is not possible to include all the work on deception and lying, these essays provide the reader with sufficient diversity to facilitate the exploration of lying in everyday life.

References

Basso, E. (1973). *The Kalapalo Indians of Central* Brazil. New York: Holt, Rinehart, and Winston.

Basso, E. (1987). *In favor of deceit: A study of tricksters in an Amazonian society.* Tucson, AZ: University of Arizona Press.

Bok, S. (1978). *Lying.* New York: Vantage Press.

Chagnon, N. (1983). *Yanomano: The fierce people* (3rd ed.). New York: Holt, Rinehart, and Winston.

Eibl-Eibesfeldt, I. (1971). *Love and hate: The natural history of behavior patterns.* New York: Holt, Rinehart, and Winston.

Foster, G. E. (1972). The anatomy of envy: a study in symbolic behavior. *Current Anthropology, 13*(2), 165–201.

Geertz, C. (1984). On the nature of anthropological understanding. In R.A. Shweder & R.A. Levine (Eds.), *Cultural theory: Essays on mind, self and emotion.* Cambridge, MA: Cambridge University Press.

Lawson, A. (1988). *Adultery.* New York: Basic Books.

Levy, R.I. (1973). *Tahitians: Mind and experience in the Society Islands.* Chicago: University of Chicago Press.

Lewis, M. (1992). *Shame, the exposed self.* New York: The Free Press.

Lewis, M., & Michalson, L. (1983). *Children's emotions and moods: Developmental theory and measurement.* New York: Plenum.

Parker, S. (1992). Personal communication, Department of Anthropology, Sonoma State University, Rohnert Park, CA.

Passin, H. (1942). Tarahumara prevarication: A problem in field method. *American Anthropologist, 44,* 235-247.

Rosin, T. (1992). Personal communication, Department of Anthropology, Sonoma State University.

Shostak, M. (1981). *Nisa: The life and words of a !Kung woman.* New York: Vintage Books.

Weiner, B., & Handel, S. J. (1985). A cognition–emotion–action sequence: Anticipated emotional consequences of causal attributions and reported communication strategy. *Developmental Psychology, 21,* 102–107.

2

What a Tangled Web:
Deception and Self-Deception in Philosophy

ROBERT C. SOLOMON

"I have done that," says my memory. "I cannot have done that," says my pride, and remains inexorable. Eventually, memory yields.
— Friedrich Nietzsche, *Beyond Good and Evil*

The average American tells 200 lies a day.
— Arsenio Hall

In this chapter, I am concerned with the connections between deception, self-deception, and our emotional engagements in the world. The prohibition against lying has occupied a central place in the history of Western ethics and philosophy, but self-deception has always been avoided as an odd, embarrassing kind of problem. Part of that problem is that self-deception and its behavioral kin, notably that "weakness of will" that the Greeks called *akrasia*, are thought to be obviously "irrational" and involve getting "carried away" or "misled" by emotion, abandoning reason and rationality. Lying and deception, on the other hand, are taken to be deliberate and clear-headed, but wicked, the very paradigm of wrongdoing. As so often in matters of mind and morals, many of the problems involving lying and self-deception can trace their origins to the classic but unfortunate dichotomy between reason and the emotions and to that even more unfortunate Manichean dichotomy between good and evil. Telling the truth is rational and good; self-deception is weakness; and deception is evil. Rejecting those dichotomies will allow us a better appreciation of the complex role of deception and the emotions in our lives.

DECEPTION IN PHILOSOPHY

Having none to recall their attention to their lives, they
rate themselves by the goodness of their opinions, and
forget how much more easily men may shew their virtue in
their talk than in their actions.
—SAMUEL JOHNSON, *Self-Deception*

Why must we have truth at any cost anyway?
—FRIEDRICH NIETZSCHE, *Beyond Good and Evil*

Throughout the history of philosophy, deception has been assumed to
be a vice, honesty a virtue. Of course, one might tactfully suggest that
the very nature of the subject, namely, the articulation of (preferably)
profound truths, requires such a commitment. If philosophers did not
seek and tell the truth, what would distinguish them from poets and
myth-makers, apart from their bad prose? Philosophers seek and tell
the truth, the *whole* truth and nothing but the truth. Or so they would
have us believe. Diogenes strolled the city looking for an honest man,
not expecting to find another but never doubting that he himself was
one. He would not have fared much better, we suspect, if he had toured
the philosophers' hall of fame. His predecessor Socrates insisted that
he was telling the truth when he claimed to know nothing, an
argumentative strategy that was doubly a lie. For many philosophers,
and scientists too, we readily recognize that the search for truth may be
something of a cover, a noble facade for working out personal
problems, pleasing parents, or pursuing personal ambition. Nietzsche
suggested that every great philosophy is "the personal confession of its
author and a kind of involuntary and unconscious memoir"
(Nietzsche, 1966). But unconscious revelation is hardly the same as
telling the truth, and some philosophers, among them Nietzsche, have
argued that there is, in fact, no truth. What have we then? Refusing to
tell the truth would then itself be a kind of truthfulness, and insisting
on the truth would be a philosophically venal sort of lie.

And yet, honesty and truth-telling have always been listed high
among the greatest virtues. Socrates, we are told, died for it. Epictetus,
the early Stoic, defended above all the principle "not to speak falsely."
In more modern times, Immanuel Kant took the prohibition against
lying as his paradigm of a "categorical imperative," the unconditioned
moral law (Kant, 1964). There could be no exceptions, not even to
save the life of a friend. Even Nietzsche took honesty to be one of his
four "cardinal" virtues, and the "existentialist" Jean-Paul Sartre

insisted that deception is a vice, perhaps indeed the ultimate vice (Sartre, 1956). Sartre argued adamantly on behalf of the "transparency" of consciousness, thus enabling him to argue (against Freud) that all deception is in some sense willful and therefore blameworthy. And today one reads American ethicists, for example, Edmund Pincoffs, who insists that dishonesty is so grievous a vice that its merits cannot even be intelligibly deliberated (Pincoffs, 1986). In this, unlike many other matters, philosophy and common sense seem to be in agreement. And whether philosophy merely follows and reports on the Zeitgeist or actually has some hand in directing it, it would be safe to say that the philosophical championing of honesty is an accurate reflection of popular morality. Lying, for philosophers and laymen alike, is wrong.

But what does it mean to insist that lying is wrong, and how wrong is it really? Is a lie told to embellish an otherwise tedious narrative just as wrong as a lie told in order to cover up a misdeed and avoid punishment? Is a lie told in desperation any less wrong than a calculated, merely convenient lie? Is a lie told out of self-deception more or less wrong than a clear-headed, tactical lie? (Is the former even a lie?) Are all lies wrong—is lying *as such* wrong—or do some lies serve an important function not only in protecting one another from harm (especially emotional harm) but in developing and protecting one's own sense of individuality and privacy? One could think of lying as diplomatic, as fortification, as essential protection for a necessarily less than candid self. Or, one could just think of honesty as merely one among many of the virtues, not a fundamental virtue at all. It is worth noting that Aristotle, in his catalog of moral virtues, lumped "truthfulness" together with "friendliness" and "wit," important traits to choose in a friend or colleague, to be sure, but hardly the cornerstone without which the entire edifice of morality would fall down. Moreover, what Aristotle meant by "truthfulness" primarily concerned the telling of one's accomplishments, "neither more nor less"—in contemporary terms, handing in an honest resumé (Aristotle, 1944). He did not seem at all concerned about social lies, "white lies" or, for that matter, even political lies except insofar as these contributed to injustice or corruption (Aristotle, 1941). Critics have often challenged Kant's analysis of honesty as a "perfect duty," appealing to our natural inclination to insist that it is far more important to save the life of a friend than it is to tell the truth to the Nazis who are after him. But if there is even one such case in which it is right to lie and honesty can be overidden, then the "perfect" status of the duty not to lie is compromised, and the question is opened to negotiation. It is in the light of such dogmatic ("a priori") condemnation too that we can understand the perennial controversy surrounding the seemingly innocent "white lie," the lie that saves instead of causing harm. And, to say the obvious (though it is often neglected by philosophers) lies can also entertain, as theater and as fiction, and not only on the stage or on the page. Indeed, lies can also be useful and fascinating in philosophy; dozens of professors are now employed because some Cretan, years ago, supposedly declared that "all Cretans are liars" and thus generated the most basic paradox in logic and philosophy. (If he told the truth, then he was lying, but if he was lying, then . . . .) Is there anything wrong with a lie when it causes no harm? And is it always true that we should tell the truth "even when it hurts?"

Behind the blanket prohibition of lying we can discern the outlines of a familiar but glorious philosophical metaphor, the truth as bright, plain and simple, standing there as the Holy Grail of Rationality, while dishonesty, on the other hand, is dark and devious, the ill-paved path to irrationality and confusion. In revealing the truth, we think of consciousness as transparent through and through; in deception we detect an opacity, an obstacle, a wall within consciousness. The honest man and the true philosopher know all and tell all (except in Socrates's case, since he insists that he does not know anything). Nevertheless, Socrates's student Plato offers to lead us out of the shadows and into the light, even at great peril. The philosopher illuminates that which the liar and the layman leave in the dark, including his or her own inner soul (Plato, 1974, VII). Truth and light are good; deception and darkness are bad or evil, leading not only to ignorance and harm but to the degradation of rationality, the abuse of language and the corruption of the soul. But philosophy, one begins to suspect, has overrated these metaphors of clarity and transparency. The obvious truth is that our simplest social relation-ships could not exist without the opaque medium of the lie.

In his novel *The Idiot*, Fyodor Dostoevski gave us a portrait of a man who had all of the virtues, including perfect honesty (Dostoevski, 1969). He was, of course, an utter disaster to everyone he encountered. More recently, Albert Camus presented us (in *The Stranger*) with an odd "anti-hero" who was also incapable of lying (Camus, 1946). It is not surprising that he comes off as something of a monster, inhuman, "with virtually no human qualities at all" (as the prosecuter points out at his trial for murder). On a more mundane and "real life" philosophical level, one cannot imagine getting through an average budget meeting or a cocktail party speaking the truth, the whole truth, and nothing but the truth. If one wished to be perverse, he or she might well hypothesize that deception, not truth, is the cement of civilization, a cement that does not so much hold us together as it safely separates us and our thoughts. We cannot imagine social intercourse without opacity. Steve Braude, a philosopher who works extensively in parapsychology, illustrates the utter importance of deception with a simple experiment. He asks his audience if anyone would take a pill (which he has supposedly invented) that would allow them to read the minds of everyone within a hundred yard radius. Not surprisingly, no one accepts the offer. We can all imagine the restless thoughts flickering through a friend's mind as we describe our latest trauma or the adventure of the day, the distracted and hardly flattering thoughts of our students as we reach the climax of the lecture two minutes before the classbell rings, the casual and not at all romantic thoughts of a lover in a moment of intimacy. "What are you thinking?" is an extremely dangerous and foolish question, inviting if not usually requiring the tactical but flatly deceptive answer, "Oh, nothing." The threatening nature of the truth has long been white-washed by philosophers (Plato and Nietzsche excepted), often under a psuedo-secularized version of the religious banner "the truth shall set you free."* But, against the philosophers, we all know that sometimes the truth hurts and the harm is not redeemed, that the truth is sometimes if not often unnecessary, that the truth complicates social arrangements, undermines collective myths, destroys relationships, incites violence and vengeance. Deception is sometimes not a vice but a social virtue, and systematic deception is an essential part of the order of the (social) world.

Now it can readily be argued that lying is just not the same thing as deception and deception is not the same thing as opacity. There is much that one may not know and may not need to know, but to be told what is not true when one asks is, nevertheless, essentially wrong, a lie and not merely deception. Deception may be nonverbal, and deception (notably in official circles) typically takes the form of a "run around" and not an explicit lie as such. There are true answers that are so misleading that one is nevertheless tempted to call them lies, and there is that protracted silence in the face of questions that even in the absence of an answer cannot be considered anything other than deception. But such complications make it much less obvious what is telling the truth and what is to count as a lie. Not to know what

---

*It is perhaps not without intentional ambiguity that this originally religious injunction (John 8:32) is engraved on the administration building of the University of Texas at Austin.

another is thinking is not the same as being intentionally misled or told what is simply not the case. It is one thing to foolishly ask, "What are you thinking?" and to be told, "Oh, nothing." It is something quite different to be told a falsehood. Evasion and deception must be distinguished, but when we look at cases, that distinction is not so neat and simple. How literal and explicit does a comment have to be to count as a lie instead of a verbal evasion. Must a lie be an answer to a specific question, whether asked or only implied? Does a lie have to be verbal at all? (We will readily admit an answer in the form of a nod of the head, for example. How about a rolling of the eyes?) Self-deception complicates this picture even more. It is one thing to self-consciously and intentionally tell what one knows to be a falsehood, but it is something quite different to tell what one sincerely believes but which turns out to be false. But what if the sincerity is superficial and one really knows the truth? Or what if one really does not seem to know but nevertheless *ought* to know the truth? The presence of that "ought" suggests that both deception and self-deception have a normative as well as a factual basis. Part of the problem is that lying seems to presuppose that one is clear about the truth oneself and then purposefully and directly misleads the other about its nature (Sartre, 1956; Fingarette, 1969). Lying, accordingly, is fully intentional and malicious, at least insofar as it willfully deprives another of something extremely important, the truth. But this presupposes a degree of rationality and transparency that just doesn't hold up to scrutiny. There are, of course, cold-blooded, self-interested lies, knowingly false answers to such direct questions as "Where were you last night?" and "Who ate all the cookies?" But one might consider the claim that such lies are the special case rather than the rule, like cold-blooded murder-for-profit in the bloody complex of accidental, negligent, desperate, and passionate homicides.

Not all lies are responses to a direct question. Not all lies presuppose knowledge. Many lies are dictated by our social roles, where truthfulness becomes a form of rebellion, and many lies are nothing more than a protection of privacy, notably "fine" as an answer to the direct question, "how are you?" Many so-called lies are not only "white" but heuristic and educational as in the various modes of fiction, the exercise of the imagination, ritual narratives and myths, perhaps even the whole of religion. Philosophers of science have long argued that the teachings of science are in an important sense fictitious, based on such useful explanatory postulates as genes, black holes, electrons, and quarks. And what of those researchers who lie and fudge data, in order to more persuasively demonstrate what they

believe to be the truth? Such "frauds" include some of the greatest
scientists in history. There are instances in which the wrongness of
lying is as straightforward as a breach of contract: "you promised to tell
me what you knew but what you told me was false." Indeed, most
straightforward lies involve some such well-defined context, a direct
question or a specific set of expectations. But our fascination with
lying and deception will not be satisfied by the straightforward case
favored by the philosophers. What we are after is a drama of truth and
falsehood in the complex social and emotional webs we weave,
compared to which what is often singled out as "the lie" tends to
become a mere epiphenomenon, an ethical "dangler" of comparatively little psychological interest.

THREE THEORIES OF LYING:
AN ELEMENTARY TAXONOMY

> To tell the truth for the sake of duty is something entirely
> different from doing so out of concern for inconvenient
> results . . . When I deviate from the principle of duty, this
> is certainly quite bad; but if I desert my prudential maxim,
> this can often be greatly to my advantage, though it is
> admittedly safer to stick to it.
> —IMMANUEL KANT, *Groundwork of the Metaphysics of Morals*

> Not that you lied to me, but that I no longer believe you,
> has shaken me.
> —FRIEDRICH NIETZSCHE, *Beyond Good and Evil*

Philosophers usually agree that lying is wrong, but they are by no
means in agreement about why lying is wrong. "Do not lie" plays a
pivotal role in philosophical disputes about ethics since ancient times.
But rather than doing a run-through of the great philosophers and
their various (sometimes remarkable) opinions, which would be
repetitive and tedious, let me summarize the issue as it currently stands
and state, rather crudely, what I think is wrong with the framework in
which these issues are typically debated. Basically, there have been
three more or less mutually antagonistic philosophical positions which
have woven their way through the literature and come to define the
current discussion. To begin with, there is the idea that "Do not lie"
has the special status of a moral law, a "categorical imperative," which
means that it is always wrong to lie, no matter what the circumstances.
In Kant's words, it is a "perfect duty," never to be excused or
overridden. "Do not lie" is, we might add, the perfect example of a

so-called "deontological" (duty-defining) principle in ethics. Lying, like breach of promise, can be argued to undermine one of the most basic human institutions, communicative speech. But lying, unlike promise-breaking, does not involve any obvious breach of a contract or pledge, and lying, unlike most other moral transgressions (e.g., theft and murder), does not as such obviously or intentionally hurt anyone. It has been argued, however, that the very nature of lying entails harm of a more insidious and pervasive nature. Every lie undermines our confidence in the veracity of speech, and at some critical point our very language will become meaningless. "Do not lie," in other words, is the perfect example for the moral imagination: "what if everyone did that?" If everyone were to lie, the answer goes, no one would believe anyone, and the very existence of language (except, perhaps, to entertain) would be threatened. And so lying is wrong in itself, not because it causes harm in any particular instance but because truth-telling is taken to be a necessary condition of our having any meaningful verbal intercourse at all.

The second major group of theorists, the utilitarians, insist that lying is wrong because a lie does, in fact, cause more harm than good. But there is no absolute prohibition here, rather perhaps a "rule of thumb," and there may well be many cases such as the infamous "white lie" in which lying causes no harm and therefore is not wrong. It may even be commendable. More sophisticated utilitarians ("rule utilitarians") offer a more thoroughgoing objection to lying by insisting that the consequences of lying *in general* (not in every particular case) weigh the balance against lying, "white lies" notwithstanding. By emphasizing rules instead of particular acts and their consequences, the "rule utilitarians" thus move closer both in temperament and in conclusions to the Kantian deontologists. Indeed, the Kantian purely hypothetical question "What if everyone were to do that?" is not so obviously different from the rule utilitarian's empirical question "What if everyone did that?" But because it focuses wholly on consequences, the utilitarian position allows and invites extensive investigative work into the more subtle and long-range effects and implications of lying, a procedure that has been well developed recently by Sisela Bok in her two books *Lying* and *Secrets* (Bok, 1978, 1984). On the basis of such investigations, she rejects means–ends arguments (such as "the end justifies the means") and upholds a virtually blanket condemnation of lying that is in practice as strict as Kant's deonotologically "perfect duty" to tell the truth.

Third and finally, there is a new contender (in fact a very old contender, promulgated at length by Aristotle) that rejects both the rigidity and centrality of moral rules and principles governing our actions and the emphasis on utilitarian consequences and instead concerns itself with the *character* of the person who performs the actions in question. What counts are not the principles according to which one behaves or the consequences of what one does but rather one's *virtues*. In contemporary ethical theory, the latest movement is the ill-named discipline of "virtue ethics" (French, 1988). "Do not lie," accordingly, becomes not a principle but an expression of a certain character trait, honesty. Moreover, the honest man is not so much one who refrains from lying, much less one who resists the temptation to lie because he or she knows that it is wrong to lie; he or she just . . . does not lie. It is built into his or her character. ("He could no more tell a lie than break the law of gravity.") Thus Aristotle insists that truthfulness must be cultivated, habitual, "second nature," and not a battle between conscience and temptation. Indeed, the intrusive presence of a "conscience" would be evidence against the successful cultivation of the virtue. Thus Dostoevski's "idiot" Prince Mishkin could not even comprehend the fact that his virtues caused catastrophe and enormous harm to other people. Camus's Meursault (in *The Stranger*) does not even understand what a lie would be, and he is declared by his author to be a kind of hero, "who refuses to lie."* This ideal of honesty as a well-cultivated virtue may seem more appealing than the usual insistence on honesty as a matter of principle or the outcome of utilitarian calculations, but it still remains to be seen why honesty should be such a virtue and why lying—not just once but habitually—constitutes a vice. Even if we make the proper distinctions and exceptions regarding lying and fiction, deception and heuristics, we need a convincing account of the viciousness of the vice. The explanation of many contemporary virtue ethicists is as vacuous as it is appealing: honesty enhances individual character, dishonesty corrupts it. But what do enhancement and corruption mean in this very individualistic context, and (just to be difficult) what is so important about enhancement and corruption of the self? Is it merely for the sake of one's self-image? What are the consequences of such enhancement and corruption of the self? Don't we know from literature if not from life that "corrupt" characters can often be charming, harmless and successful? Aristotle, who restricts his

---

*Albert Camus, *The Stranger* (New York: Random House 1942). Camus's commentary on his novel was published over a decade later, in the preface to Germaine Greer's 1955 edition. Camus's judgment is compromised by the fact that Meursault does lie in the novel, indeed, commits outright perjury, and his obliviousness to matters of morals make it highly unlikely that he can be said to "refuse to lie."

discussion to truthfulness regarding one's accomplishments, suggests that truthfulness is the "mean between the extremes" of boastfulness and mock modesty. But this does not seem to provide the account we are looking for, which would require something more than social impropriety or mere obnoxiousness. On behalf of Aristotle, one might argue that his answer is already presupposed in the social framework of his ethics, not just in the sense that the "right amount" of truthfulness would be a matter of shared agreement among his aristocratic peers but in the more currently agreeable sense that truthfulness like all virtues becomes a virtue and gains its significance only within a social context in which people are inextricably tied together in their pursuit of the good life. Truthfulness is a personal virtue not just because it is good for the individual soul but because it is to some extent essential to the well-being of the community as a whole.

What gets left out of the three standard accounts is what Aristotle takes for granted: the effect of lying and deception (also self-deception) in interpersonal relationships. As Nietzsche so wisely complains, in characteristic opposition to Kant, "Not that you lied to me, but that I no longer believe you, has shaken me" (Nietzsche, 1966). It is not the breach of principle against lying that is so troublesome, nor is it the consequences of a lie which might in themselves be wholly benign. Nor is it that the character of the liar is necessarily compromised or impugned (he or she may already be a rotter) but rather that his or her relationships are compromised, corrupted. The problem, here as elsewhere in philosophy, is that lying is not taken seriously as a *social* phenomenon, a way that people interact. The standard philosophical emphasis on principles, consequences, and the isolated concept of individual character deemphasizes or even ignores social relations and relationships between particular people (as opposed, for example, to the general notions of "the public good" or "society.") Of course, any philosophical theory worthy of the name will be sufficiently flexible to claim to encompass and include such personal and social implications, whether as part of the preconditions of the theory or by way of subtle and extended calculation (as, for example, an economist might claim to explain all of human behavior by way of "cost/benefit" analysis and utility maximization). The problem is not that social and personal relations cannot be included in such theories but rather that they are sidelined, deemphasized, reduced at best to mere "instances." But the thesis I want to pursue here is that the wrongness of lying does not have to do primarily with breaches of principle or miscalculations of utility, even if these weigh heavily in particular cases—in a court of law or congressional hearing, for example. Lying is wrong because it constitutes a breach of *trust*, which is not a principle but a very particular and personal relationship between people (Thomas, 1989).

Neither is the wrongness of lying primarily a matter of "character," although, to be sure, questions of character and integrity do arise, not so much in the relationship itself as when one steps back to reconsider, "sizing up" one's friend or colleague anew in light of a recent deception or betrayal. Furthermore, one might argue that this concept of character is at best probabalistic and not deterministic. It allows us at most a tentative summary of what an individual has done and a prediction based on less than perfect knowledge about what he or she will probably do in the near future. And, of course, this notion of character tends to ignore or make light of those all-important "out-of-character" performances, and it also neglects that important dimension of "will power" or "resolve" so celebrated by many of the existentialists, notably Sartre (Sartre, 1956). The problem with the emphasis on character in most virtue ethicists is that it does not get at the intricacies of human relationships, the way different traits are expressed and stimulated (or inhibited) when two or more people get together. Virtue ethics presupposes a measure of psychological autonomy and constancy of character that is probably implausible, in part, one surmises, because of moral philosophy's obsession with talking about more or less isolated ("autonomous") individuals and the equally misleading tendency to talk about relations with *strangers*, or "someone or other" rather than friends or family or lovers. Social interchange may be presupposed and implied in any discussion of the virtues (one cannot be "generous" or "charming" if there is no one else to give to or to charm), but it is not the social dynamic itself that gets highlighted in current studies of virtue. In traditional philosophical ethical theories, notably in deontology and utilitarianism, the dynamic and the social nature of ongoing activities and relationships typically gets ignored in favor of what Pincoffs rightly calls "quandary ethics," an emphasis on particularly difficult situations and dilemmas (Pincoffs, 1986). But shifting that focus from situations and the principles that govern them to the character of the individual does not recapture the lost social dynamics that have been so long ignored or neglected or dismissed as mere "psychology" by philosophers. Lying is, essentially, a social activity. It not only involves other people (which is obvious) but is part of the intercourse that binds people together. Thus, lies to strangers are a peripheral concern. Official lies by politicians and professional lies by doctors and others in positions of authority are a special case. Lying is first of all a matter of interpersonal trust, and to say that lying is wrong is to point out that a lie breaches the very trust it necessarily presupposes, not in the abstract sense argued by Kant but in the very personal and concrete sense that usually goes by the name of "betrayal."

Is it, therefore, always wrong to lie? The question here is not the "perfect" nature of the imperative not to lie nor is it a cost/benefit analysis according to which most lies are harmful and a few "white" lies may be harmless. If lying is first of all a matter of breaching the trust of a relationship, it follows that the severity of the lie depends on the nature of the relationship and the understanding that forms that trust. This is by no means a simple matter. There are relationships that are built on a lie, relationships that thrive on lying, relationships in which only the participants know where the truth begins and ends, and relationships where uncertainty and not trust as such is the glue that holds them together. There are willing suspensions of trust which presuppose an underlying trust in turn, explicitly in the case of fictional storytelling and performances of various kinds, tacitly in the case of the "sore spots" in any relationship where deception may be the better part of valor. No, lying is not always wrong, and the seemingly simple difference between right and wrong becomes rightly muddled once we appreciate the personal rather than the abstract moral implications of lying.

SELF, DECEPTION, AND SELF-DECEPTION

The difficulty making such distinctions [between real and only apparent truthfulness] is almost as great for liars as for their dupes, because self-deception enters into such estimates to such an extraordinary degree. Hypocrites half believe their own stories, and sentimentality makes fraud take on the most innocuous tints.
—Sisela Bok, *Lying*

You're a liar, like most people. You lie to yourself.
—Elia Kazan, *The Arrangement*

Self-deception is also a dynamic social phenomenon, not just an internal drama or a pathological condition. The "social" nature of the phenomenon, however, is often less than obvious, but part of the reason for this is that philosophers tend to think of self-deception as an odd and even paradoxical version of deception, as a "lie to oneself," not involving other people in any way at all. Of course, the lie may well be "about" other people—as in a lover's self-deceptive vision of his or her beloved, and other people may be *affected* by one's self-deception, as they themselves are deceived in turn. But a conception of self-deception that begins with the idea that the dynamics of self-deception are self-contained will lose the essential thread, which is not merely terminological, between deception and self-deception, namely, their shared role in our social and personal relationships. So, too, it is important to get away from the static "knowing and not knowing" conception that characterizes many philosophical studies of self-deception (Audi, 1988). As an integral part of an ongoing relationship both deception and self-deception are necessarily dynamic, unstable (or, perhaps, "metastable"*) and a continuous effort of enormous complexity (Sartre; 1956; cf. Baron, 1988).

Deception and self-deception, I want to argue, are conceptually distinct but thoroughly entangled phenomena. Superficially, one essentially involves other people, the other does not. But to treat them as different versions of the same phenomenon in two very different settings or to treat them wholly differently (as lying and lying to oneself, respectively) to is to miss the dynamic that motivates both. To fool ourselves, we must either fool or exclude others; and to successfully fool others, we best fool ourselves. Philosophical discussions of lying too often take as the paradigm example the straightforwardly cynical, self-interested lie and ignore the more common species of lying that is in part self-deception as well. Transparency to ourselves can be just as intolerable as transparency to others and for just the same reason. The self, with all of its flaws and failings, is all too evident. The recognition of one's own motives and the significance of one's own thoughts can be devastating to one's self-image and sense of self. Part of the self is self-presentation and self-disclosure, but an aspect of equal importance is the need to hide, not to disclose, those facets of the self that are less than flattering, humiliating, or simply irrelevant to the social context or interpersonal project at hand. But the self is essentially a social construct, and our sense of ourselves depends on other people, or what Jean-Paul Sartre called (with just a touch of paranoia) "our Being-for-Others" (Sartre, 1956). One can hide or refuse to disclose oneself to oneself in many ways, notably by ignoring or distracting oneself. Epictetus, while

---

*A term that Jean-Paul Sartre borrows from chemistry in his mammoth *Being and Nothingness*. Metastability has a tentative stability, an appearance of stability, but the slightest intrusion or misstep brings about toal disaster. Consider a waiter carrying an overly full tray of cups of hot coffee. All goes smoothly until the first jiggle, and a single boiling hot drop touches his bare skin. He flinches slightly, and . . .

defending the principle "not to speak falsely," complained at length about those philosophers who, instead of applying the principle, went on and on about abstract "meta"-questions and simply ignored the truths to be told. One might hesitate to call this evasion self-deception (although it often leads to and, more importantly, stems from self-deception), and it would surely be unfair to call philosophers "liars" just because they prefer to avoid the truth and talk about truth instead. But what philosophers do (more or less for a living) is what all of us do some of the time, namely, distance ourselves from ourselves and *rationalize*, that is, use the truth insofar as it furthers our ambitions and embellish it as needed when it does not. Thus, Samuel Johnson (1987) wrote, of self-deceptive men who would be virtuous, "Having none to recall their attention to their lives, they rate themselves by the goodness of their opinions, and forget how much more easily men may shew their virtue in their talk than in their actions." Thus deception and self-deception are intimately intertwined. We fool ourselves in order to fool others, and we fool others in order to fool ourselves. And to make it more complicated (as it should be), we do not always know which is which, who is self, and who is other.

Deception between persons is rarely so cynical that it does not involve more than a trace of sincerity and belief, in most cases the belief that even if this particular "fact" is false, the truth that the lie is protecting is far more significant than the act of lying. Thus we have the lover who lies to protect his love, or the scientist who fudges her results to "prove" a hypothesis she just "knows" to be true. Sisela Bok rightly suggests that there is a thin line at best separating the lie for the sake of the truth and the lie that marks one a liar. Lying for the sake of the truth is a paradox that already requires a considerable amount of self-deception. Deception between persons is rarely if ever unmotivated, and even a mischievous lie "for its own sake" (the familiar "shaving" of one's age, for example) is typically a cover-up for other lies, insecurities, and distrust. As we start to understand deception and self-deception as an essential aspect of self-consciousness and not as a willful violation of principle or antisocial act we begin to lose that sense of blanket condemnation of "lying as wrong" and understand deception and self-deception as part of the matrix of human relations, neither good nor evil as such but open to sympathy and understanding rather than blame. People tell lies not only to avoid punishment or to impress others but because they need to protect themselves (their selves) and cope with difficult social situations. Within the limited realm of self-knowledge, in particular, deception is almost always a matter of coping rather than a celebration of falsehood as such. Indeed, what it means to be false to oneself is a rather complex ethical problem; our knowledge of ourselves is not only incomplete but undergoing continuous revision, often along the lines of ideals and ambitions that are themselves ill-conceived, inappropriate, or merely borrowed. It is within this continuing authorship of self and self-esteem that both deception and self-deception must be appreciated, and even the most cynical interpersonal intrigues are first of all shared productions of the self, involving both conspiracy and vulnerability in more or less equal measure. Consider, for example, the web of affections and deceptions in Chodoros Laclos' *Liasons dangereuses*, which deceptively presents itself to us as an aristocratic game but soon reveals itself as a life-or-death theater of mutual self-deception. And as in *Liasons dangereuses*, (whose author felt it necessary to produce a lengthy preface morally denouncing and distancing himself from the psychology he so insightfully represented), what is too often presented as a morality tale becomes a study in interpersonal psychology and the mutual, partly hidden, surreptitious construction of the self (Laclos, 1962). It is not as if ethics is (or should be) absent from such a study, but our evaluations can no longer be of the Manichean "truth is good, deception is evil" variety.

Even in the most straightforward cases, where neither deception nor self-deception is an issue, telling the truth is not always a virtue. One can use the truth as a weapon and honesty as a strategy. Children and lovers, as authors on the subject often point out, frequently tell the truth precisely in order to hurt and to humiliate. Truth-telling can be manipulative, even vicious, and a conscientious ethicist might well question whether this ought to count as the virtue of truth-telling, even if the truth is being told. (If not, might not its opposite, refusing to tell the truth in order not to hurt, be counted a virtue?) In Camus's novel *The Fall*,* an extremely devious character named Clamence confesses to an acquaintance (the reader, of course) the truth about his life, including first and foremost the many lies he had always been telling himself (Camus, 1956). What becomes obvious, however, is that he is still deceiving himself by way of seducing the other, and even his truths are only a ploy. What Clamence is after, we come to learn in the last pages, is not truth or total disclosure but a subtle vengeance, and his confession is a subversive expression of a deeply felt resentment. But who is the victim, and who is the villain, in such

---

*In many ways the opposite of *The Stranger*. Meursault (the "stranger") is the very portrait of transparency, all experience and virtually no reflection or self-consiousness. Clamence, by contrast, is all reflection and painful self-consciousness. One tells the truth because he is too simple-minded to lie, the other because he wants to seduce his listeners. In what sense is either of them "not lying?"

tales of deviousness? It is an appreciation of the truth, after all, that makes the strategy so effective. And why do we think that victims and villains must be part of the structure of deception? As often as not, deception and self-deception combine to form the most sincere belief. Virtually every faith and religion is a large scale example of such belief, but so too is almost everyone's self-image and every society's sense of itself, including the scientific and philosophical communities as well as every ethnic group or culture. Nietzsche and, later, Jung wrote extensively on our need for myths and warned against an age that would try to do without them. But what is a myth if not an elaborate self-defining collective self-deception, and if all such deceptions are wrong then would there be any truth that is ultimately worth defending?

If deception and self-deception are to be understood first of all as interrelated dynamic interpersonal and social phenomena, then it is a mistake to try to understand them in terms of one or another artificially isolated aspect of the relationship. For example, in most modern discussions of lying, much of the focus has been on the alleged victim, the person who is misled or betrayed by the lie. The evaluation thus tends to trace out the obvious and not so obvious effects of even the "whitest" lie, its ability to undermine trust and render the victim helpless when the truth might well have allowed some significant action. Sisela Bok, for example, pursues such a quest in wonderful detail, tracing the consequences of professional lies, political lies, loving lies, paternalistic lies, therapeutic lies, experimental lies, etc. (Bok, 1978). Bok discusses at length the complications of authoritarian deception and the manufacture of excuses, including the notorious "slippery slope" argument from the very plausible claim that "the whole truth" is impossible to tell down to the insidious thesis that the truth is not necessary. That is the challenge and the fun of philosophical investigations of lying, of course; first we recognize the obvious immediate consequences: hurt feelings, a tragically un- or ill-informed patient (client, friend, public). Then the devastating penalties for an unsuccessful "cover-up" become evident. Finally, there are the more subtle implications of spreading distrust, increased cynicism and consequent withdrawal, a corruption of language and public discourse. What gets left out of many of those discussions of deception, however, is the need to focus on the liar and not just the consequences facing the liar. For if deception and self-deception are so intimately involved, then the assumption that the perpetrator of the lie is not also its victim becomes less plausible. The lie is a matter of mutual engagement and not just a malevolent act perpetrated by one person upon another.

Alternatively, when philosophers have fixed their gaze on the nature of the lie instead of its consequences they have tended to even further deny the interpersonal and social nature of deception. Kant in particular was adamant about the logical inconsistency of the "maxim" of any and every lie, established by the fact that one could not universalize the allowability of lying without undermining the very possibility of language (assuming, that is, that the primary purpose of language centers around such activities as describing true facts and making promises) (Kant, 1964). Of course, because lying is (by definition) the *intentional* telling of a falsehood, some attention must be focussed on the liar who has and exercises that intention. But Kant quite explicitly dismisses and ignores the motives and the character who lies behind the lie, preferring to emphasize the immorality of lying rather than to understand the psychological and social dynamics. But even as ethics, it is certainly not unimportant to identify what motivates lying and what kind of characters we are dealing with when we point our fingers at liars. Here is where "virtue ethics" gains its hold. But to overemphasize the character of the liar is just as misleading as an isolated emphasis on the lie or its consequences. Deception is, to employ an overused and much abused word, a *holistic* phenomenon. One cannot break it up into parts and expect to understand its vital organic unity. One cannot try to understand or evaluate the lie, the liar, the victim, and the consequences and then put these together in some "multidimensional" analysis which adds up to an adequate understanding.

One of the most distinctive and most neglected features of lying is that it is surprisingly hard to do. As anyone who has tried to protect even a small casual lie can tell you, the amount of thought and care that is required to keep in mind all of the logical implications and possible contradictions ("If I was at Sam's place, then I couldn't have seen Thelma at the Casino, but if I didn't see Thelma then how could I have known about the party at Shelby's house?"). It is always easiest, the old adage tells us (with considerable truth), to tell the truth. But next easiest is to believe your own lie, to become so submerged in its network of details and implications that the continuation of the lie—as Aristotle argued for honesty—becomes but second nature, without further thought or deliberation. In either case, however, neither ease nor difficulty is a dependable mark of morality, and one might (like a novelist or any other story teller) delight in the intrigue and self-conscious tension that artful lying requires. Part of the pathology of compulsive liars may well be the high-adrenalin challenge of holding a number of lies together as a high-risk acrobat might juggle a number of brightly-lit torches or razor-sharp knives—

along with the sometimes psychotic need to cover up not just something but (by logical implication) almost everything. Here, of course, there is some temptation to scissor off the liar from any particular lie or any particular audience, but a moment's reflection makes it clear that this too is a distinctively and often compulsively public performance, part of a possibly rich and probably very deep pattern of self-deception as well as a way of relating to other people, despite the fact that the nature of the relationship may be quite puzzling or offensive to them. So, too, with more innocent and straightforwardly strategic lies. Lying involves a complex logic that reaches across and cuts through our various social relationships and sometimes with great difficulty weaves a portrait of the self and its relations. And even in self-deception, it is the inconsistencies in our stories discovered or discoverable by other people that motivate our continued efforts at duplicity. After all, if self-deception were a matter of mere internal consistency, would anyone but a logician feel compelled to avoid inconsistency at all costs? Would "cognitive dissonance" ever become an issue much less a motivational force if it did not also become subject to the scrutiny of others (Festinger, 1957)?

No matter what the challenge or the logical complexity of the lie or the effects of the lie on the liar and his or her social entanglements, the primary concern always seems to be the benign or harmful effects of the lie on the listener. But here again there is a social matrix and a set of interpersonal presumptions that generally go unnoticed. What renders most lies odious is that they occur in a context in which one expects the truth, most obviously, in response to a direct inquiry. But even there the odiousness of the lie depends on the context and the nature of the question ("What are you thinking?") and there are circumstances in which only a Kantian or a paranoid would insist that the truth is essential and lying immoral. Imagine yourself on an intercity bus or a short-hop plane ride next to a somewhat tedious fellow passenger who insists on asking "What do you do?" One can readily imagine offering up the most banal and boring answer as an alternative to an utterly offensive reply, or, alternatively, one can with slightly more effort imagine constructing a fascinating but wholly false account of one's life as a K.G.B. double agent or a Texas Ranger. In the first case, one gets a chance to get some reading or sleeping done, while in the second, there would seem to be no harm done but rather a welcome entertainment for both of you during an otherwise tedious voyage. There is, of course, the odd chance that one's fellow passenger may (contrary to all expectations) show up again, wreaking the sort of havoc that only fans of old movies can fully appreciate, and it is true, no doubt, that every lie opens one up to possible complications of this sort. But this is hardly a moral objection to lying, and in the absence of harm such elaborate lies seem unobjectionable. (So, too, one could argue, for the "big lies" that hold most religions and cultures together.) But here again the attention should be on the social context and the relationship—in the above case essentially transient—and not on the lie or the consequences of the lie exclusively.

In the preceding section ("Three Theories of Lying"), I complained that not only the limited emphasis on the logic of the lie and its consequences but excessive concern for the character of the liar ignores or minimizes the importance of the social and interpersonal context. To see this, it would be worth our while to ask how it is that lying corrodes the character of the liar. One obvious suggestion is that lying becomes a habit. But the habit of lying is not like biting one's fingernails or mindlessly repeating some inessential figure of speech or sound when nervous. Lying, even self-deception, requires thought and keen self-awareness. One does not lie unknowingly, unconsciously or by accident, as one might bite a fingernail or insert "you know" in every other sentence. Indeed, one might well argue that an accidental lie is no longer a lie. If I tell you that the cookies are in the cookie jar, but meanwhile Sally has eaten them all, I am not lying. I am just wrong. If I unthinkingly utter a falsehood—perhaps after waking from a dream or being absorbed in a book—I can hardly be properly accused of lying.

Lying is not corrupting just because it becomes habitual. But it may nevertheless be true that every time one lies one makes lying a little easier. First of all, "practice makes perfect," and by practicing lying one learns to prepare better lies and better protected lies. Having to follow through the logical vicissitudes and implications of a seemingly simple falsehood is remarkably invigorating intellectual exercise, and though this might be a dangerous pedagogical technique for those of us who teach still malleable adolescents, any improvement in one's intellectual acuity will at the same time improve one's ability to tell a successful lie. But, of course, improving one's ability to lie need not and usually does not increase one's propensity to lie, and why should increasing expertise mark moral degeneracy? Improving one's marksmanship does not make one a murderer and studying locksmanship does not render one a burglar. A better suggestion still is that practice in lying brings about a certain callousness toward the truth, a loss of qualms about lying. Paul Ekman writes that children are very hesitant about telling a first lie ("should I or shouldn't I?") but "after that, [they] lose the ability to consider it" (Ekman, 1990). Against this, however, one should compare the findings of Michael Lewis (this volume, Chapter 4).

Children begin their careers in deception not by lying but by play-acting, by feigning, by living in a world of stories and scenarios in which truth and fiction are not yet delineated and in which lying is therefore not yet an option. Indeed, children are sometimes shocked to be chastised for "lying" when in fact they have only been relating one or another feature of their undifferentiated world-view which their elders designate as false rather than as fantasy. Thus, one typically begins to lie not out of calculation or in one's own self-interest, and the discovery that lying can be an important tool in the arsenal of one's egoism is itself a considerable contribution to one's moral degeneracy, quite apart from any actual acts of lying that may follow. But this suggests that the questions of character that concern the virtue ethicist are indeed not questions about the corruption wrought by any particular action or sequence of actions but pieces of a much larger picture of an overly self-interested person for whom lying is but a single and not easily differentiated aspect of an already manipulative selfishness. It is not that lying corrupts character so much as the fact that lying is a sign or symptom of corruption and that corruption can best be described as a deficient sense of relationships with others. The truth is but one of the many victims of violated trust and willful manipulation.

From an interpersonal and social perspective on deception and self-deception, we can begin to get a clue about the philosophical tendency to isolate the lie and the liar and ignore the personal relationships in which lies play their role and, sometimes, wreak their damage. So, too, we can understand the more general tendency to declare, in uncompromising terms, the sheer *wrongness* of lying. It is much easier and far more comfortable to analyze the logic of lying and moralize about withholding or hiding the truth than it is to accept our own complicity in the world of deception and self-deception. What bothers us most about lying, to put it bluntly, are *other people's* lies. And so we go out of our way to explain why lying, in general, is wrong, conveniently forgetting about or rationalizing as something other than deception our own not infrequent liberties with the truth. The condemnation of lying is itself a part of a social matrix, a harsh expression of one's own desire not to be the victim of a lie. Just as the lie is segregated as a particularly vicious bit of perverted verbal behavior, liars are isolated as a particularly perverse sort of character. It is often hypothesized, for example, that lying represents deep insecurity, antisocial behavior, and low self-esteem. But it would at least be worth noting the very different observation, that learning to lie may be a critical feature of growing up and developing as an individual. Children's lies are, of course, a parent's nightmare, indicating a loss of immediate access and the consequent loss of control. But these lies also represent independence, the individualization and individuation of consciousness. One learns of the intimacy and privacy of one's own thoughts not through a Cartesian soliloquy but by deceiving other people, if only by answering "Nothing" to the intrusive question, "What are you thinking?" One discovers that one's thoughts and feelings are one's own when one finds out that, with a certain amount of effort and skill, they can be kept a secret. Lying thus supplies a mechanism for selfhood and marks off the separation of one consciousness from another. It provides the means of protecting one's private thoughts and forbidden fantasies.

Self-deception further reinforces individuality by supplying the unrealistic dreams and fantasies that allow a person to cope and thrive in difficult or even impossible circumstances. But self-deception like deception has its origins not in juvenile incipient criminality but in the undifferentiated self-conception that emerges in the child only belatedly in words and self-descriptions. One might misleadingly argue on this basis (as some religious thinkers have argued) that all self-conception is ultimately self-deception, that there is no "self" as such and that all self-conceptions constitute a dangerous illusion. But a more common sense description of the same evolutionary chain would be that the self emerges never fully-formed from a murky complex of tacit and only sometimes articulate self-images and self-reflections; that self-deception is nothing other than a slightly misleading name for the inconsistencies and familiar flaws in the attempted integration of the self. Naturally, we are disturbed and offended by these flaws in other people and the lies they tell us in order to protect and project themselves. But no matter how moral we may be, we have either fewer qualms or a more generous understanding of our own complicity in the world of deception, for we understand how essential it is to our very existence as individuals.

Thus it is a mistake to think about and condemn deception and self-deception *sui generis*. Not only are there legitimate lies in literature, heuristics in science, myth in religion and philosophy, but these are not just isolated fictional frames from which considerations of self and others are excluded. Quite the contrary, these are the "myths and metaphors we live by," according to many authors from the ancients to our contemporaries. Once we give up the philosophical tendency to generalize about deception and self-deception in the abstract and focus instead on the particular lie, the intentions and motives behind it, the context as well as the consequences and the interpersonal relationship between the participants, it becomes increasingly obvious that most lies are not merely lies but also self-deception and part of a larger matrix of beliefs and emotions that define not only this relationship but a community or a culture. The lies of love (or pretended love) depend for their credibility on a remarkable institution that defines and gives structure as well as elaborate discourse to a seemingly "primitive" emotion (Barthes, 1977). Consider how much cultural apparatus goes into the simple but vicious lie, when someone falsely utters "I love you." And how often is such a lie uttered in fact with the knowledge or at least a host of doubts that it is or may be a lie? Self-deception, like deception, is motivated not by self-interest, cold and calculating, but by our engagement in an emotionally charged world in which things *matter* to us, and matter more to us than that abstract meta-conception known to us as "the Truth." Deception and self-deception are part and parcel of our engagements in the world including, not least, the development and maintenance of our image and sense of ourselves. Deception is first of all a way of relating, to others and to oneself. Some deception is harmful and even immoral, but some of it is neither. Indeed, an extremist might argue that there is no such phenomenon as lying as such, only various ways in which we relate to one another as peculiar creatures surrounded and infiltrated by language. We are, perhaps, not only capable of lying but virtually incapable of not doing so (Nietzsche, 1979; Baudrillard, 1988). Deception and self-deception, according to such a kinky view, may not be perversions so much as they are the very stuff of human intercourse.

PHONY FEELINGS:
THREE FORMS OF EMOTIONAL DECEPTION

> We are only undeceived
> Of that which deceiving could no longer harm.
> —T. S. Eliot

Why do we deceive ourselves and others? Typically, we deceive one another and ourselves to protect our emotions and our emotional attachments. We deceive one another and ourselves because of our emotions and our emotional attachments. We deceive one another and ourselves within our emotions and our emotional attachments. One can read Freud as a paranoid rationalist: in self-deception we defend ourselves *against* our passions. Sartre, on the other hand, suggests that we defend ourselves *through* our passions (Sartre, 1938).

But both Freud and Sartre turn out to be rationalists of a similar stripe, playing off the emotions against the clarity of reason and the ideal of a transparent conscious, with nothing to hide. For Freud, such a transparent conscious is impossible, of course, but it is the theme of virtually all of Sartre's plays and novels (e.g., *No Exit* and *The Condemned of Altoona*). In those plays, the transparent rationality of consciousness gets clouded if not obliterated by such emotions as fear, pride and shame, but the ideal remains in tact nevertheless. Where Freud sees emotions as psychogenetic obstacles to clear-headed self-consciousness, Sartre sees them as devices we willfully use to distract ourselves. But, ultimately, the two positions are not all that different, in that they share a lack of appreciation for the emotions and the enormous complexity they involve (Solomon, 1981).

We talk, ambiguously, of "false" emotions. Sometimes, of course, an emotion might be said to be false just because one has the facts wrong, but, because an emotion is "subjective" (that is, it depends on the beliefs of the subject rather than the facts of the case as such), an emotion may be "true" even if the facts of the case later show it to be unwarranted. What is much more revealing are the relationships between an emotion and its expression and between an emotion and its motive. Just as the expression of an emotion may be inappropriate even where the emotion itself is perfectly proper, an emotion may be absent when its expression is obligatory (e.g., at a funeral or at a wedding). We hesitate to call such emotional pretense "false," but only because we understand the ritualistic context in which such performances are required. Where the context does not demand such a performance and we do not believe that the person has the emotion expressed, we do not hesitate to call him or her a "phony," a fraud. But if philosophers in their obsession with reason and valid arguments do not pay enough attention to emotions in general, they certainly do not pay enough attention to the vicissitudes in self-deception. To be sure, even Plato and Aristotle worried about the fact that emotions interfere with reason and rational argument and thus play a causal role in self-deception and other irrational behavior, but neither they nor very many philosophers since have attended to the complexity of self-deception within the life of the emotions, not as "irrationality" but, at least sometimes, as a desperate attempt to make the world make sense. Thus the hallmark of self-deception is *rationalization*. It is not a form of irrationality but an attempt to make the world rational.

Self-deception, and deception in general, must be motivated. Just as telling a falsehood does not count as lying if the speaker does not know the falsity of his or her statement, neither is a statement that is not intended to deceive but does so (perhaps because the listener does not understand it or is himself self-deceived). So, too, in self-deception it is not enough that a person holds two contradictory beliefs and is (or seems to be) unaware of one of them; that lack of awareness must itself be motivated (Gur, 1979). It is important to emphasize that to insist that deception and self-deception are motivated is not to say that the motive in question must be essentially selfish. It need not be one's own self-interest that is at stake, much less calculated self-interest, and one's interests need not be antagonistic or inconsiderate toward others; indeed, one's motivation may be precisely their interests. (Parental self-deception about children and the infatuation of the lover for the beloved are the most obvious examples.) Motivation involves much more than tiny tugs of greed; it also embraces the way we see, take part in, and respond to our world. But mainly, our motivation in everyday social life consists mainly of emotion (desire, I would want to argue, is vastly overrated), and it is the emotions that determine much if not most of what we call "character" and thus determine the face we put forward to others. Not surprisingly, vain and wishful creatures that we are, we therefore aspire to and insist on certain emotions rather than others, depending on our circumstances, and when we do not actually have the emotions that we think that we "ought" to have, we may manufacture them. When an emotion is manufactured, however, it may be that the resulting emotion is nevertheless the genuine article. Sometimes, the resultant emotion or emotional display is half-hearted, unconvincing, or downright fraudulent. These are the "phony feelings," and I want to distinguish and outline three different varieties of them.

The first is straightforward pretense, a form of deception but not self-deception. One acts as if one had an emotion but does not (or one pretends to have an emotion other than the one he or she actually has). One of several complications, however, is that one cannot pretend in a vacuum, and the circumstances and story must be "appropriate," no matter how accomplished one's acting talents. Moreover, as William James pointed out a century ago, pretending to have an emotion is often the best way of actually coming to have that emotion, and pretense thus turns into real emotion. Sisela Bok notes in a footnote that the word "hypocrisy" originally derived from the Greek word for "answer," as employed by actors on the stage (Bok, 1978). She then goes on in the text, "Hypocrites half believe their own stories, and sentimentality makes fraud take on the most innocuous tints." Here again is that crucial linkage between deception and self-deception, facilitated by emotion. ("Sentimentality" is much too limited.) Accordingly, great actors sometimes put themselves "inside" of the character they wish to play, which means taking as their own the character's emotions and concerns. The more they come to actually feel and believe this, the more effectively they will play the role. But while feigned feelings are certainly "phony," whether appropriate or not, they do not yet constitute full-blown emotional self-deception.

The second form of deception regarding emotion is self-deception, but self-deception *about* one's emotions, denying that one is angry when one is obviously furious, for example, or fooling oneself into thinking that he or she is in love, when in fact the emotion in question is of a very different nature. Again, there are fascinating complications, for insofar as emotions are (at least in part) cognitions, the judgments we make about our emotions have logical connections with our emotions. What we think we feel is therefore not unrelated to what we actually do feel. Deceiving ourselves about the emotions we feel is obviously tied to the different values we place on the various emotions and the way self-esteem rides or suffers, not so much from the fact that one has a certain emotion but from one's acknowledgment that one has it. Thus people who feel deep resentment or envy will typically identify those unattractive emotions as "hate" or "contempt." Shamed school-boys deny their fear and instead insist (implausibly) that they were angry. Disappointed lovers redefine their love as infatuation or, more demeaning, mere curiosity. Emotions mark status. In an elitist society, contempt is thought to be a noble emotion. In a romantic society (let's not leap to the self-deceptive conclusion that we are one), love will mark stature, while in a competitive society pride will be promoted while jealousy is provoked. An emotion which is glorified and encouraged in one culture is feared or despised in another. A litigious society such as our own will praise anger and indignation, while a more stoical society of Eskimos will condemn such emotions as "childish" (Briggs, 1981). We have a considerable investment, therefore, in what emotions we have and are seen to have. It is extremely foolish therapeutic advice, therefore, to insist that one should "simply accept one's feelings, without judgment." What one accepts and refuses to accept in the realm of his or her feelings is itself an essential constituent of a self-conscious self-identity.

It is the third form of deception that I find the most fascinating and also the most neglected. It is also a form of emotional self-deception, but it consists of deception *within* the emotions and not in our judgments about our emotion. The two forms of self-deception often accompany one another and conceptually play off against one another but, nevertheless, must be distinguished. The key to this third form of deception, once again, is the cognitive nature of emotions. Emotions, as cognitions, can go wrong in a variety of ways. They may be based on mistaken information. They may be based on faulty inferences or insufficient evidence. They may involve spurious claims or unjustified evaluations. And as we can and do deceive ourselves about what we believe, so, too, we can and do deceive ourselves in those beliefs and judgments that constitute our emotions.

Simply getting the facts wrong is not, as we commented above, sufficient to make an emotion "phony." But there are "self-deceptive emotions," emotions that undergo what psychoanalysts call transference and the related property of the "detachability" of an emotion from its proper context (deSousa, 1988). Thus a female patient might fall "madly" in love with her analyst, deSousa tells us, "regardless of the latter's loveableness." Emotions can also be phony, according to deSousa, by internalizing an ideology, a politically manipulative set of beliefs. A woman's frustrated guilt when she ought to be angry is the product of an ideology in which women are not entitled to be angry, and a man's jealousy, deSousa suggests, may presuppose an ideologically founded assertion of property rights. I have some doubts about these examples but not about the overall strategy they employ. It is a mistake to think that self-deception can only take place on the level of fully conscious articulated beliefs (the model that gives rise to the paradoxes discussed above). There is also the strategic manipulation of our perceptions and judgments on an inarticulate (not to say "subconscious") level, systematic refractions or distortions that attempt to constitute the world and the self in a more comfortable way. But whether conscious and articulate or inarticulate and unnoticed, our emotions can be seriously distorted by circumstances and by ideas which may well become self-destructive. Moreover, self-deceptive emotions (like self-deception in general) have a "rippling effect"; they have "to expand [their] boundaries to be efficacious" (Baron, 1988). Thus a self-deceptive emotion will not be self-contained, one flawed passion floating through consciousness oblivious to the psychological flux that surrounds it. Self-deceptive emotions corrupt what Baron calls "our belief-forming processes," and as a result we gradually rationalize our situation, reinforce our own bad habits, and turn to blaming others, cementing ourselves not just in a matrix of fraudulent emotions but a way of life that is most likely fraudulent as well.

It has long been suggested (e.g., by Leibniz back in the seventeenth century, by the Stoics thirteen centuries before that) that our emotions are "distorted" perceptions or judgments, that *all* emotions are, in this sense, self-deceptive. To pick but one obvious example, *love* has often been lampooned or criticized for its willful self-deceptions, for its exaggerating out of all reasonable proportion the charms and virtues of one (rather ordinary) person, for its utter obliviousness to obvious evidence, for its boundless wishful thinking. But is this a fair example, and is love indeed an example of pervasive self-deception? The intricacies of this question would take us far beyond the already bloated scope of this essay, but a few words on the genuineness of emotion are surely in order here. Are all emotions indeed self-deceptive (as rationalists of every age have often argued)?

Every emotion structures the world according to its own distinctive categories. In anger, the world (or someone or some act in it) is offensive; in jealousy and fear, the world is threatening; in love, one's beloved is "lovable." Is this a distortion? Of what? Of that cold, impersonal view of the world that scientists and philosophers have too often held up as their ideal—devoid of values and attachments except as items for study? Of some more or less "objective" viewpoint adopted by people who do not care or are not involved? Of course, someone who does not see an act as an offense will neither get angry nor see the point of anger, and one who does not find another attractive, charming, or lovable will neither fall in love nor comprehend someone else's doing so (except perhaps with the throw-away line, "there's no accounting for tastes"). But it is perversity to evaluate those judgments which presuppose engagement by standards that exclude any involvement or attachment. It is now a cliché that "beauty is in the eye of the beholder," which may be untrue of art but seems to be certainly true of love. Of course, in retrospect (when the love is over) one may well look back and judge that he or she was mistaken about the supposed virtues of the once beloved, but this no more undermines the validity of the judgment than does the irrelevant opinion of a third party casual observer. Emotions are not, as such, distorted or "self-deceptive," although they can be, like any complex psychological phenomenon through which we gain our sense of self and self-identity. But self-deception, like deception, has its limits, set by the context and the presuppositions it may well take for granted. And among those presuppositions is our confidence in the general validity of our emotions, a confidence which two-and-a-half thousand years of philosophy have not yet successfully undermined.

References

Aristotle (1944). *Nicomachean Ethics* (trans. W. D. Ross). Oxford: Clarendon.

Aristotle (1941). *Politics* (trans. B. Jowett). In R. McKeon (Ed.), *The works of Aristotle*. New York: Random House.

Audi, R. (1988). Self-Deception, rationalization, and reasons for acting. In B. McLaughlin & A. Rorty (Eds.), *Perspectives on self-deception*. Los Angeles: University of California Press.

Baron, M. (1988). What is wrong with self-deception? In B. McLaughlin &

A. Rorty (Eds.), *Perspectives on self-deception*. Los Angeles: University of California Press.

Barthes, R. (1977). *A lover's discourse*. New York: Farrar, Straus and Giroux.

Baudrillard, J. (1988). *Selected writings*. Palo Alto: Stanford University Press.

Bok, S. (1978). *Lying: Moral choice in public and private life*. New York: Random House.

Bok, S. (1983). *Secrets*. New York: Random House.

Briggs, J. (1981). *Never in anger*. Cambridge, MA: Harvard University Press.

Camus, A. (1946). *The stranger*. New York: Random House.

Camus, A. (1956). *The fall*. New York: Random House.

deSousa, R. (1988). *The rationality of emotions*. Cambridge, MA: M.I.T. Press.

Dostoevski, F. (1969). *The idiot* (trans. Henry & Olga Carlisle). New York: New American Library.

Ekman, P. (1990). *Why kids lie*. New York: Scribner.

Festinger, L. (1957). *Cognitive dissonance*. Evanston, IL: Row Peterson.

Fingarette, H. (1969). *Self-deception*. New York: Humanities Press.

French, P. (Ed.) (1988). *Ethical theory: Character and virtue*. Notre Dame: University of Notre Dame Press.

Freud, S. (1929). *Standard edition of the collected works*. London: Hogarth.

Gur, R. C., & Sackheim, H. A. (1979). Self-deception: A concept in search of a phenomenon. *Journal of Personality and Social Psychology, 37*(2).

Johnson, S. (1987). Self-deception. In C. Sommers (Ed.), *Virtue and vice*. San Diego: Harcourt Brace Jovanovich.

Kant, I. (1964). *Groundwork of the metaphysics of morals* (trans. H. J. Paton). New York: Harper Torchbooks.

Kazan, E. (1974). *The arrangement*. New York: Avon Books.

Laclos, C. (1962). *Liaisons dangereuses*. New York: Penguin.

Lakoff, G., & Johnson, M. (1980). *Myths we live by*. Chicago: University of Chicago Press.

Martin, M. W. (1986). *Self-deception and morality*. Lawrence, KS: University Press of Kansas)

McLaughlin, B. B., & Rorty, A. (Eds.) (1988). *Perspectives on self-deception*. Los Angeles: University of California Press.

Nietzsche, F. (1979). Truth and lying in the extra-moral sense. In *Philosophy and truth* (trans. D. Breazeale). Atlantic Highlands, NY: Humanities Press.

Nietzsche, F. (1966). *Beyond good and evil* (trans. W. Kaufmann). New York: Random House.

Pincoffs, E. (1986). *Quandaries and virtues*. Lawrence, KS: University Press of Kansas.

Plato (1974). *Republic* (trans. G. M. A. Grube). Indianapolis: Hackett.

Rorty, A. (1972). Belief and self-deception. *Inquiry, 15*(winter), 387–410.

Rorty, A. (1980). Self-deception, akrasia and irrationality. *Social Science Information, 19*, 905–922 (reprinted in McLaughlin and Rorty, 1988).

Sartre, J. -P. (1938). *The emotions*. New York: Philosophical Library.

Sartre, J. -P. (1956). *Etre et l'neant* (trans. as *Being and Nothingness* by Hazel Barnes). New York: Philosophical Library.

Solomon, R. C. (1976). *The passions.* New York: Doubleday-Anchor and Notre Dame: University of Notre Dame Press.

Solomon, R. C. (1981). Sartre on emotions. In P. Schilpp (Ed.), *The philosophy of Jean-Paul Sartre.* London: Open Court.

Thomas, L. (1989). *Living morally.* Philadelphia: Temple University Press.

3
Animals as Liars:
The Human Face of
Nonhuman Duplicity

ROBERT W. MITCHELL

ANIMALS AND DECEPTION

> Dogs show what may be fairly called a sense of humour. . .;
> if a bit of stick or other such object be thrown to one, he
> will often carry it away for a short distance; and then
> squatting down with it on the ground close before him, will
> wait until his master comes quite close to take it away. The
> dog will then seize it and rush away in triumph, repeating
> the same manoeuvre, and evidently enjoying the practical
> joke.
>
> —CHARLES DARWIN, 1871

Perhaps more than any other of their activities, deception by animals persuades us that we are dealing with an entity which, however different in appearance, is similar to humans psychologically. Like people, animals know how to manipulate us and their conspecifics, and we respond to their manipulations by endowing them with complex intentions and desires. Yet when animals' deceptive behaviors are examined more closely, we sometimes find less evidence of psychological complexity than was at first apparent. At other times, we find that characterizations like Darwin's are not so far off.

Whereas observers such as Darwin in the nineteenth and early twentieth centuries viewed humans and nonhumans as psychologically similar, later observers became somewhat more reticent about making such assumptions. No doubt this reticence stemmed from the historically earlier dismissal of the need for any psychological explanation for the suitability of organisms to their situations, a dismissal that developed from Darwin's theory of natural selection. Before Darwin's (1859) *Origin of Species*, most Western scientists and

59

intellectuals believed that nonhuman activities resulted from the intentional intervention of a mindful deity not unlike a human agent. Any intelligent activities an animal displayed (such as deception) were evidence of this deity's design. Darwin's theory of natural selection effectively countered this argument for design by offering an account which did not require a designing deity, but the theory also had the effect of making any psychological inferences from animal behavior increasingly suspect and consequently avoided by many scientists.

Yet animals' deceptions still have the power to draw us in, much as a mirror entices us to look—we are often more interested than not when we see a bit of ourselves in someone. Animal deceptions engage our attention, if only via anthropomorphic pretense. The ease with which we extend human qualities to nonhumans suggests, however, that our anthropomorphism may be more than just pretense; that in fact some animals' deceptions are psychologically like our own. Perhaps, to understand nonhuman deception, it would pay not a little to first understand human deception.

When Lipmann and Plaut published their 1927 German-language book *Die Lüge* which presented (according to its full title) "the lie viewed from the standpoints of psychology, philosophy, jurisprudence, pedagogy, history, sociology, philology and literature, and developmental psychology," the only chapter to discuss deception by nonhumans was Alverdez's (1927) "Deception and Lying in the Animal Kingdom." In this chapter, I take much the same position as Alverdez, in presenting the range and complexity of deception by many species in a book largely devoted to detailing the range and complexity of deception by one species. To fulfill my task, I first discuss the nature of human deception, and suggest that pretense is essential to its nature. Next I define deception and hiding, as well as camouflage and distraction, and then develop a hierarchy of levels of psychological and other processes which lead to deception and hiding, in which each level builds upon processes present in lower levels, and examine evidence of animal activities which suggest attainment of a particular level. Using this hierarchy, I attempt to disentangle nonhuman deceptions which involve pretense, planning, and knowledge of other minds from those based upon simpler processes.

HUMAN DECEPTION AND PRETENSE

It is perhaps no coincidence that most definitions of pretense do not distinguish it from intentional deception. Like mature deception, pretense is simulative or "as if" behavior. Yet pretense is not a constituent of all deceptions. What deception and pretense share, at a metaphorical level, is the "doubleness" of their referents: they appear to be one thing, but actually are another. But in some cases the relationship between deception and pretense is more than metaphorical, because in these cases deception entails pretense.

Pretense, as such, implies a psychological description. According to Walton (1990), when engaging in pretense participants imagine themselves to be actually enacting the activities which they are only pretending to enact. They are engaging in a game of make-believe, in which it is fictional that they are really doing something. If they are pretending to be cops and robbers, then they are fictional cops and robbers—it is fictionally true of them that they are cops and robbers—and they imagine themselves accordingly. The player's actions are *representations* of robbing, ambushing, arresting, and so forth, which means that their actions function as props in a game of make-believe. These props prescribe imaginings of a particular sort—those which have to do with cops and robbers. The objects that they use to further their pretense, such as the sticks which serve as guns, are also props in their game of make-believe. Pretend activities may simulate quite closely activities in a real situation—"You are under arrest" may be said in both instances, for example—but even when pretend and real activities are identical, the pretend actions are supposed to be recognized as *representations* of the real activities.

The distinction between make-believe and reality is, in Walton's view, understood by the pretender, even though this understanding may be outside immediate awareness. Apparently, even 2-year-olds distinguish pretense from reality (Leslie, 1988): they can sip tea from a cup filled with tea, and they can pretend to sip tea from an empty cup. However, recognition of pretense as such in humans seems rather labile, especially for very young children (Harris, 1989). For such cognitively immature creatures, the psychological marker which distinguishes fictional from nonfictional reality is, at times, easily forgotten. On one occasion, while playing with 22-month-old twins, I pretended to be a monster. Although initially both boys pretended to be afraid, yet smiled on running back to be captured by the monster, for one of the boys I eventually became a "real" monster: he stood apart staring fearfully, moaning slightly, and clasping his hands looking for reassurance, while his brother continued to run back and forth. Even at three years of age, a child can confuse his own rendition of a monster with the "real" thing (DiLalla & Watson, 1988). Such inadvertent failures to retain the recognition of pretense suggest that the fictional reality of the pretense can come to be experienced as literally real. The boundaries between fantasy and reality may become clear quite early (at 5–6 years old) when the fantasy is not based on real events. But older children can also become so immersed in a pretense that they lose sight of the distinction between reality and pretense. When pretending to have an imaginary playmate, children seem to be of two minds about their playmate, wavering between a belief in its reality and a recognition of it as part of their game of make-believe (Singer & Singer, 1990). Even adults can become so engaged with their pretense and fantasy that they respond to them as to reality. One woman who accurately feared that her husband was having an affair engaged in pretense to avoid confronting her fears: "I made up a lot of excuses, and really believed them...I didn't confide in anyone, too, because I was afraid of what they would tell me" (Werth & Flaherty, 1986). Such knowledge of the pretense in the midst of denial of this knowledge is self-deception, a topic of some import discussed below.

The labile shifting between fictional and literal reality derives from the nature of the experience of pretense. We often experience our pretense as really happening; thus, it is easy to get caught up in the world of our pretense, even though we begin with an awareness that it is not real. How often the adult finds him- or herself believing, if only momentarily, what was only a daydream! Because the experienced reality of the fictional world of pretense is so engrossing, the distinction between the fictional and real worlds is sometimes lost, even after the knowledge of pretense is fairly well in place.

Ontogenetically the enacting of pretense leads to the ability to plan—to imagine oneself engaging in courses of events. Indeed, a plan is an imaginal (pretend) scenario or narrative in which a series of events occurs in the mind of the imaginer, with the recognition that the scenario is imaginal but could be (or is going to be) enacted by the imaginer. Planning to have events take place in pretend play begins at about 2 years of age (McCune-Nicolich, 1981). Imagining oneself in situations other than the present one can work in at least two ways: one could imagine oneself in a situation and then attempt to create that situation (as in planning and pretense), or one could imagine oneself in a situation and then avoid dealing with the correspondence between that situation and reality (as in pretense and self-deception).

To summarize, then: pretense involves representations, which are props that promote or inspire a particular game of make-believe. This game of make-believe is typically organized according to a scenario, and elements of the scenario are sometimes decided beforehand. The props need not stand for anything that is real: monsters and unicorns can be represented as easily as cops and robbers. The game of make-believe is experienced as real or literally true while also marked as fictional, such that the game is, fictionally, really true. Sometimes this experienced reality (marked as fictional or pretend) can be so engaging that the fictionality marker is ignored or denied and the pretender believes that the pretend experience is, in fact, real—the player pretends that the pretense is reality, knowing all along that it is pretend.

Pretense, Deception, and Self-Deception

This characterization of pretense is more than reminiscent of intentional deception. Just as in a mutual pretense, the objective of intentional deception is to enact a particular scenario and thereby build up particular beliefs congruent with this scenario in one's own and the other's mind. Just as in pretense, the scenario is marked for the deceiver as fictional or pretend, which means that the deceiver experiences the deception as fictionally true. Deception from the deceiver's point of view can be thought of as a game that the participant "plays along with" while not really believing. But just as in pretense, the deceiver sometimes experiences the scenario as literally true, even while knowing that it is a deception; and sometimes victims of deception also recognize the deception but simultaneously continue to believe the falsehood, engaging in a self-deceptive game of make-believe in which they deny the fictionality of the fiction prescribed by the deceiver (Werth & Flaherty, 1986).

Initially, self-deception from the self-deceiver's point of view seems different from pretense. Although the self-deceiver can be thought of as "playing a game," the game is one that the person denies participating in, even when confronted with contrary facts (Graham, 1986). However, when the experience of self-deception is examined, it seems to involve an initial acknowledgment of the contrary facts, followed by a denial of their relevance (Werth & Flaherty, 1986). I suggest what happens during the self-deception is that the person's acknowledgment of the contrary facts leads to the following: (1) the beliefs that the person desires to believe are marked as fictional or pretend—and are thus believed to be, fictionally, really true—while (2) the contrary facts and the marking itself are denied or ignored—hidden from view—because they do not fit in with the storyline of the pretense. Pretense thus serves as a basis for self-deception.

As in any pretense, in self-deception we ignore information not relevant to the ideas currently being used. Also as in pretense, the desired beliefs are repeatedly acknowledged and the contrary beliefs ignored. But in self-deception the person feels a resulting discomfiture because of the experienced inconsistency of his or her beliefs (Graham, 1986; Werth & Flaherty, 1986). The person experiences the "desired" beliefs as true, even while recognizing that they are fictionally true, in much the same way that one experiences passages in a good novel as true, even while recognizing that the passages are fictionally true. The recognition of the beliefs as fictionally true is implied in the self-deceiver's feelings of disturbance when she experiences as inadequate or exaggerated the excuses and explanations invented to account for the contrary facts. The self-deceiver imagines him or herself in a particular scenario and "plays along" with this scenario. The imagined scenario is a *representation* of what the self-deceiver wishes were the real situation; it is a prop in the self-deceiver's game of make-believe.

The line of argument presented in this section should encourage the beliefs that pretense is a substrate for intentional deception as well as for self-deception, and that both intentional deception and self-deception are types of pretense. Deception differs from a mutual game of make-believe only in that the "partner" (the deceiver hopes) is unaware of the pretense. The deceiver can appear sincere because the pretense is sanctioned within the game of make-believe played by the deceiver. The victim is caught in the same game of make-believe, but does not recognize it as such.

DEFINITIONS

Pretense is, however, part of only some deceptions: many deceptions occur without any imagination at all. Metaphorically at least, mimicries of plants and insects are as much deceptions as are planful manipulation by humans. Such metaphorical similarity means that there is an underlying structure which encompasses these phenomena. It is this underlying structure to which I wish to give definition.

It is surprising to think that a definition exists which could satisfactorily include every instance of deception ranging from mimicry to intentional deception. It becomes even more surprising when one recognizes the extent of deception in living organisms: the biological world is filled with deception. Mimicries alone are classifiable into at least 18 types with multiple subtypes and numerous (and in some cases apparently innumerable) distinct instances of each (Pasteur, 1982), nonhuman primates offer several types of non-mimetic behavioral deceptions (de Waal, 1986; Whiten & Byrne,

1988) which permeate their day-to-day lives, and human deceptions are so myriad that classification seems inexhaustible. To tie together the many instances of deception, I offer the following definition of deception (based on and elaborated from Mitchell, 1986), designating the organism to be deceived as the "victim." Deception occurs when the victim registers or perceives, from the deceiver, something (the "prop") which simulates or represents something else (the "sign"); the sign influences (or would influence) the victim to do or believe something, which is an appropriate response to the sign for the victim; the victim responds to the prop as to the sign; the function of the sign for the deceiver is to influence the victim to do or believe what the sign would make the victim do or believe; and such a response by the victim is inappropriate given what is actually the case. Note that self-deception is incorporated in this definition when deceiver and victim are the same organism.

Camouflage is not covered by this definition because its function is to *avoid* having something be registered by the victim; camouflage is only effective if the victim does *not* notice the hidden organism. As a result, although camouflage is often considered a type of deception, it is more usefully thought of as the reverse of deception. In camouflage, the camouflaged organism benefits when the victim *fails* to register the camouflaged organism because it is (designed to be) indistinguishable from something which is without significance to the victim. Camouflage blends into deception in some instances, however: insect larvae that look like bird droppings, for example, may be registered by a bird and interpreted as unworthy of attention (in which case the larvae *deceives* the bird), or the bird may simply not notice the larvae at all (in which case the larvae is *camouflaged* from the bird). When the victim takes a camouflaged organism to *be* something, the camouflaged organism deceives; when the victim does not register the camouflaged organism, the camouflaged organism does not deceive. So the same "disguise" may serve two functions. Similarly, a person dressed up to look like someone else both deceives as to his or her identity and hides (camouflages) his or her real identity. Camouflage occurs when a camouflager, or some part or product of the camouflager, has an attribute which simulates something that would be, or is, unlikely to be registered or attended to by the victim; and the function of the attribute for the camouflager is to make the victim fail to register that which has the attribute.

Not all hidings are camouflages, although all camouflages are hidings of a sort. Hiding occurs when the hider has some attribute and/or achieves some effect, the function of which is to make the hider (or some product of the hider) inaccessible to the registrations of a victim. There are innumerable ways the attribute or effect can make inaccessible the victim's registration of the hider or one of its products, depending upon the perceptual systems of the victim. The effect might be countershading and positioning of the hider such that it blends into its surroundings; or it might be transforming the medium in which the victim perceives, as an octopus does when it sprays ink into the water to cover its escape. The attribute might be a chemical which makes the hider olfactorily indistinguishable for the victim from members of the victim's own species. Contrary information which is being denied in self-deception is also hiding of a sort.

An activity midway between deception and hiding is distraction (see Whiten & Byrne, 1988). Distraction occurs when the distractor does something, the function of which is to cause the victim to be inattentive to something else, where the victim's inattentiveness allows the distractor to do something which it could not do if the victim were attentive. Monkeys distract a mother by grooming her so as to be close enough to kidnap her infant without interference (Hrdy, 1979), and people distract a dog they are playing with by petting it until it loosens its grip on an object, or by pointing away from an object in front of the dog to divert its attention, so that the person can get the object from the dog (Mitchell & Thompson, 1991). Distraction implies a two-part process: the distractor first gets the other to fail to register something, and then the distractor, aided by the other's failure to register, does something which reveals a secondary motivation. Although in many instances the distracting activity simulates or represents another activity (and hence utilizes deception), in others the activity simply causes the victim's attention to lapse or be redirected without deceptive means (as when the groomed monkey mother or the petted dog lapses into inattentiveness). Sometimes people attempt to distract themselves from attending to bad news (thus, the distractor is the victim, as in self-deception), and nonhumans appear to do similar things when they "feign interest" in something apparently uninteresting to avoid attending to something unpleasant or disturbing (de Waal, 1986).

PSYCHOLOGIES OF DECEPTION AND HIDING

Note that the definitions of deception, camouflage, hiding, and distraction make reference to registration or inattentiveness by the victim. As we shall see, even when deception and hiding are designed by evolution and natural selection, the perceptual (registrational) processes of the victim are necessary for their creation (Mitchell, 1986). Yet it seems obvious that the deceptions and hidings of humans differ in their psychology from those of dogs, and that both of these differ from the deceptions and hidings of butterflies. To allow for meaningful discussion of the different types of deceptive activities, I propose a hierachy (derived from Mitchell, 1986, 1987, 1990, in press-a) which describes subsumptive levels of these activities. In this hierarchy are six levels of processes of increasing complexity which create different forms of deception, hiding, and distraction. Processes at the lowest level are evolution, selection, morphogenesis, and registration by an observer (the victim). The second level adds the registrations of the agent (the deceiver) coordinated with actions of the agent. The third level adds learning and memory. The fourth level adds pretense and, consequently, abilities for self-awareness (conscious thought) and imaginative planning. The fifth level adds taking the other's perspective. And the sixth level adds recognizing the other's perspective on the self's perspective. In this hierarchy, higher-level processes retain aspects of lower-level processes, such that, for example, planning (which is a higher-level process) requires that one be capable of learning and perception (which are lower-level processes). This framework offers insight into the *types* of mental processes which can vary among organisms of different species and which are necessary to develop to the point where one can gain mutual understanding.

Selective Registrations

Deception at the first two levels (many described in Edmunds, 1974, and Owen, 1980) encompasses what is commonly called mimicry or camouflage, but these levels differ in the involvement of the agent. At the first level are simulations, produced through selection, evolution, and morphogenesis, which were selected for their resemblance, from the victim's perspective, to things that have special relevance (mimicry) or no relevance (camouflage) to the victim. The victim's registrations, then, are an active selective agent, as Darwin (1859) noted. These first-level resemblances require no action on the part of the deceiver. Everyday examples of first-level deception are the viceroy butterfly which looks like the unpalatable monarch butterfly to birds which learn to avoid both, and the butterfly whose wing-tips look like a head and antennae to predators which bite these and thereby afford the butterfly escape. Even plants produce deceptive mimics: to stop butterflies whose caterpillars eat the plants they reside on from laying their eggs on the plant, the ends of its leaves and tendrils simulate eggs of the butterfly. Plants also produce first-level camouflage, as when they simulate pebbles or dead vegetation to avoid visually guided predation. Some animals hide from predators by living concealed in an enclosure. Others, such as caterpillars of swallowtail butterflies, look like bird droppings on the top of leaves. In all of these instances, the victim's registrations, but not the deceiver's registrations, are involved in the production of the deception.

Mimicry at the second level differs from the first in that the mimetic resemblances require registration by the deceiver (or hider) for the deception to be put into effect. One striking example of second-level deception is the eyespots exhibited by innumerable insects and even a species of frog. When these animals are attacked, they expose or make salient parts of their body which resemble eyes, thereby scaring the attacker. The eyespots are only revealed when the animal detects a predator or is otherwise disturbed. Sometimes this second-level deception is coordinated with first-level camouflage to avoid predation: the peacock butterfly, for example, looks like a dead leaf when at rest with its wings closed, but when disturbed its wings open and close with a hissing sound, revealing and hiding four large eyespots. Some animals feign death when disturbed; some snakes, for example, produce a particularly elaborate death-feigning display, wriggling about uncontrollably and ending with their mouth open and tongue hanging out. Predatory fireflies mimic the reproductive flash patterns of fireflies of another species to capture them; birds feign injury to lead predators away from their nest; and molting stomatopods (a type of shrimp) whose cavities are invaded by other stomatopods mimic their own display which bluffs their willingness to fight even when they are incapable of inflicting injury (see Mitchell & Thompson, 1986). Distraction appears to enter the hierarchy in many deceptions at the second level; a nondeceptive instance suggested by Wickler (1968) is the tail-waving of cats, lions, lizards, and snakes, which distracts the prey while the predator attacks. Olfactory disguise occurs in the beetle which exudes chemicals mimicking those of different ant species so that it can move comfortably through their colony without harrassment (Vander Meer & Wojcik, 1982); and acoustic hiding is present in the silence created by hunting predators. Cephalopods such as octopus and squid hide behind an inky screen which they propel from their body when confronted by a predator (Moynihan, 1985). Camouflage used by cephalopods and other creatures which match their environment to hide from predators is also second-level hiding, because they must register things in their environment to effect the change.

Learning And Memory

Third-level deceptions and hidings go beyond mimicry to produce resemblances which are not specifically or solely designed by natural selection in concert with the registrations and actions of deceiver and victim alike, but which require the additional processes of learning and, consequently, memory for their existence. The addition of learning does not insulate the organism from its evolutionary history or from its own or another's registrations. Instead, an organism's learning is constrained by these processes, such that animals are more likely to be affected by some stimuli over others. For example, if Krebs' (1977) Beau Geste hypothesis is correct, birds which are genetically programmed to imitate the diverse repertoires of numerous avian species do so because their expanded repertoires suggest what appears to be a crowded environment to other birds, who are thereby dissuaded from nesting nearby. Here we see clearly the influence of selection on learning propensities, but selection can also produce organisms whose learning is much more open to environmental influences. That is, we might expect some organisms which are particularly attentive to the influence of their activities upon their social and physical world to have a selective advantage over others not so gifted. These organisms would be expected to notice that when they enacted a particular action, a particular result typically followed; the resulting predictive ability is the basis of instrumental conditioning. (The significance which many deceptions have for victims of deception is similarly acquired through learning—see Wickler, 1968; Quiatt, 1984; Mitchell, 1986; Mitchell & Thompson, 1986.) Learned deceptions, then, would range from functional deceptions in which the animal had no knowledge of the underlying relation between the benefit it achieves and its behavior, to intentional actions in which the organism predicts the functional relation between its deceptive actions and their resulting benefits. However, at this level the animal has no knowledge of how its victim interprets these misleading actions, and so the actions are not intentionally *deceptive*, however much the animal intends to perform them.

More sophisticated third-level deceptions suggest that the animal learns to perform some action in order to effect some consequence. For example, animals such as dogs and chimps which have received attention as a result of an injury sometimes limp as though injured to gain sympathy (de Waal, 1986; Goodall, 1986). Learning to *control* behaviors also leads to deception and hiding. One common deception requiring such control is object-keepaway, the mammalian play project of moving toward the partner with an object only to move the object away when the partner attempts to obtain it (Mitchell & Thompson, 1991). This play project may develop from the animal's controlling its retrieval. For example, a puppy began to play object-keepaway only after its retrievals of a ball to its owners continually resulted in loss of the ball (Mitchell, 1990). Another example of deception based on control is a captive elephant which avoided an aggressive encounter by acting as though to turn on a shower for another elephant, which caused that elephant to move away from the deceiver and toward the shower (Morris, 1986). And a captive gorilla enjoyed startling people who were watching her as she pounded the window of her cage; because people habituated to her repetitive window poundings, she began to fake window slams to keep people attentive (Quiatt, 1984). The incompleteness of the deceptive actions of the puppy, elephant, and gorilla indicates their ability to control their activities.

Presumably animals that can learn to effect a result by performing or controlling particular actions can also learn to *avoid* a result by *not* performing particular actions. Children often stop themselves from expressing their feelings because they recognize the social conse-quences of that expression (Saarni, 1989). Chimpanzees on hunting raids learn to control noisy expression of their emotions and therefore hide acoustically from prey more effectively (Goodall, 1986). Chim-panzees also sometimes look at something which seems unimportant to hide embarrassment, and rhesus monkeys act as though they have not noticed mild threats from dominant monkeys because the dominant monkey will not respond to the lack of response (de Waal, 1986). Two captive elephants camouflaged their stealing of hay by unobtrusively swinging their trunks apparently aimlessly—one from side-to-side, the other from front-to-back —as they moved to pick up and retrieve hay from other elephants' haystacks (Morris, 1986). The same gorilla who faked window poundings to keep people's attention also acted as though indifferent to people's response by looking at things other than the people, while still watching them peripherally before her window slams and fake slams (Quiatt, 1984). Learning to control some activi-ties may occur rapidly: after waiting until other chimpanzees had left, one chimpanzee barked loudly upon receiving bananas from observers at Gombe, which caused the others to return and take his bananas; the next day he again waited, but this time he emitted only faint sounds upon receipt of the bananas (Goodall, 1986).

Many animals, then, manipulate others' actions by their own actions. In some cases, these manipulative activities appear to have been planned by the animal. An example of apparently planned behavior was observed in Peter Ashley's dog (described in Dennett, 1978). One evening this dog whimpered for Ashley to get out of the only chair she was allowed to sleep in, but Ashley remained there. The dog left Ashley and scratched at the door to be let out. When Ashley got to the door, the dog ran to the chair Ashley had just left. (Jeannette Ward, a knowledgeable and experienced comparative psychologist and breeder of Wiemaraners, informed me that one of her dogs sometimes barked while looking out the window to get other dogs off the couch so that she could lie down.) Dennett suggests that only knowledge of act–response contingency is necessary to understand this deceptive distraction: the dog believes that when she scratches the door Ashley moves to the door, so she scratches. However, the explanation is insufficient: if the example is to be believed the dog embedded her knowledge of the person's response to her door scratching into her desire to get into the chair, such that the dog believed that she could get into the chair if she scratched the door to get Ashley out of the chair (see Russow, 1986). My point is not to argue that Ashley's dog had this belief (she may have desired to go for a walk and then noticed the chair was empty when Ashley made it to the door), but to indicate that, if she had this belief, she was able to incorporate her understanding of the contingent effects of her own actions into a plan along the lines of "If I do X, he will do Y, and then I can do Z" (see de Waal, 1986). Such an "XYZ plan" is not very elaborate, but would entail the dog's imagining what she could do to get Ashley off the chair.

One problem with interpreting the dog's deception as the result of a plan is that we do not know anything about past contingencies between the dog's activities and the person's responses. Because we do not know how the dog came to understand these contingencies, we cannot reasonably expect to understand the dog's knowledge of them. Misinterpretation might occur whenever we choose to interpret the end-product in the development of a behavioral sequence without reference to its development. For example, in a study by Mason and Hollis (1962) a rhesus monkey A learned to use the behavior of another monkey B to decide which of four carts to choose. Monkey B saw which cart contained food, whereas monkey A did not; if monkey A chose the cart containing food, both monkeys received food; otherwise, neither monkey received food. Monkey A learned to pull a ring to make monkey B visible and then used monkey B's behavior to decide which cart to choose. This depiction suggests that the first monkey planned along the lines of "If I make the informant visible, he will help me decide which cart to choose, and then I can get the food." But this pattern appeared only gradually, suggesting that the mental representation which developed was not formulated in advance by the monkey. The trial-and-error nature of the learning of the rhesus monkeys in this and other tasks, and the failure of a particularly savvy pigtail macaque to formulate an XYZ plan, the effectiveness of which was made to be salient (Silverman, 1986), suggest that these monkeys and others like them come to deceive via learning rather than planning.

XYZ plans seem more common in apes than in monkeys (see de Waal, 1986; Miles, 1986). For example, during my first meeting with the sign-using orangutan Chantek, he distracted me to get raisins and nuts he had seen me put into my pocket. While touching me from the opposite side of a fence, he looked at me and then slowly turned his head to my left; as I turned to see what he was looking at, he put his hand in my pocket to obtain the food. In the absence of other knowledge about Chantek, it is difficult to interpret his actions psychologically. His distraction suggests planning ("If I look this way, he'll look this way, and then I can get the nuts"), but may have resulted from a gradual history of trial-and-error learning. Either way, I was totally taken in.

Pretending to Be Another and Planning

Must we remain skeptical of any implication of planning on the part of an animal? Obviously we need to devise experiments to disentangle the various explanations for an animal's behavior, but I think that coherent theories of an animal's psychology can be derived from knowledge of multiple aspects of that animal's developmental history (Köhler, 1925; Birch, 1945; Piaget, 1947). In particular, I suggest that an animal that plans should also evidence pretense of others' actions, because planning has an imaginal component which is concomitant with pretense of others: both involve kinesthetic-visual matching (Mitchell, in press-a, in press-b). To pretend to be another, one must recognize that one's own actions, usually experienced kinesthetically, are the same as those of another, experienced visually. Both planning and pretending to be another indicate an agility at imaginal representation which can be used to manipulate others.

The fourth level begins with the ability to pretend at another's actions and, consequently, to plan. The learning present at the third level is required for the fourth level, in that the planner must be able to anticipate the outcomes of its actions. Given that imaginal pretense is necessary for intentional deception, organisms should exhibit evidence of pretending to be another before we can assume that their deceptions are intentionally deceptive. Even if one is overly generous in attribution of pretense, observations of pretend play among nonhumans raised among conspecifics are exceedingly rare. Indeed, the only nonhumans so far observed to engage "naturally" in pretense of another are rhesus monkeys and chimpanzees, and the incidents are so few as to seem questionable. On Cayo Santiago, one rhesus monkey used a coconut shell as a prop representing an infant carried by her mother: the monkey, holding the coconut shell in the same position as her mother held her infant, followed her mother about, shifting placement of the coconut shell to mirror the mother's placement of the infant (Breuggeman, 1973). At Gombe, chimpanzees enacted nonsocial pretenses: lone chimpanzees enacted aggressive displays on three occasions; one chimpanzee repeatedly imitated another chimp's aggressive display with a kerosene can; and one chimpanzee imitated her mother's ant-fishing, but to "an imaginary nest" of ants (Goodall, 1986). In contrast, once they have interacted extensively with people, the pretend play of some nonhumans is elaborate and shows a surprising similarity with human pretense (see Mitchell, 1987, 1990): the home-reared chimp Viki pretended to have an imaginary pulltoy, which, as with imaginary figures in human children (Singer & Singer, 1990), ended when someone participated directly in the fantasy; sign-trained chimpanzee Washoe, gorilla Koko, and orangutan Chantek all played with dolls and seemed to attribute psychological qualities to them; and, much as young children imitate their parent at work, dolphins imitated the work of divers cleaning their tank, using a variety of objects as algae scrapers and emitting a stream of bubbles similar to those of the divers.

In all these instances of nonhuman play, support for their interpretation as pretense derives either from the apparent substitution of one object for another or from the animal's apparent interpretation of nothing as something; that is, the animal's activities imply that the animal is using a thing (or nothing) to *represent* something. The characterizations are most questionable when the animal uses nothing to represent something. Yet these same characterizations are very appealing as evidence of complex psychological experience. Of the solitary aggressive displays by Gombe chimpanzees, Goodall asks "Who are we to say that these actions were not performed expressly to terrorize a host of imaginary chimpanzees?" Of the chimp imitating her mother's ant-fishing, she asks, "[H]ow do we know that [her twig] was not swarming with a record, though nonexistent, catch?" Goodall's questions suggest that their answer is unknowable, so we had best opt for pretense. But why not opt for hallucination, or some genetic factor which compels the organism to imitate and practice aggressive displays and termite fishing? Is there any compelling evidence to distinguish among pretense, hallucination, or ritualization to explain these behaviors? Goodall's questions raise more than just the issue of pretense in chimpanzees. What about the apparent pretense in the normal play of nonhumans? Do animals engaging in playfighting, for example, imagine that they are, fictionally, really fighting?

This question has plagued researchers of nonhuman play for decades. An early researcher of play, Groos (1898), wondered about the extent of pretense in nonhuman play. Groos described pretense as "conscious self-deception," suggesting that the motivation for playful imitation is that the organism is pretending or imagining that it is really doing what it is imitating. He noted that play simulates other functional activities, and believed that some nonhumans recognize the simulation as such. For play to be pretense Groos required this recognition, which would be evidenced by the play activities being a (nonidentical) imitation of *another's* enactment of the real behaviors which the play represents. Bateson (1955) similarly evaluated animal play for pretense. For Bateson, if a playing organism or its partner recognizes the resemblance between play and nonplay activities, then the play activities refer to the nonplay activities; animals playfighting would be, fictionally, fighting, just as children playing cops and robbers are, fictionally, cops and robbers (see Mitchell, 1990, 1991a).

Against such an analysis is the argument that simulative actions in play are designed by natural selection (i.e., ritualized), and thus involve no *intentional* simulation. Although playfighting resembles fighting, the argument goes, playfighting animals are not pretending because they are not intending to produce simulations of fighting— their playfighting actions do not *represent* fighting, in Walton's terminology, they just look like fighting to human observers. Still, there are suggestions that some nonhumans, specifically rhesus monkeys (Breuggeman, 1978), can indeed represent fighting in their playfighting (though it becomes a question whether they *always* do), such that the playfighting acts as teasing or implies a threat. These monkeys enact playfighting to bully or thwart a monkey while hiding their veiled threat from other monkeys which might interfere. If this interpretation is correct, it means that monkeys can indeed recognize the impact of their own ritualized behaviors and can detach themselves from these behaviors to use them for their own ends. The animal is not pretending to be another, but may instead be pretending about its own actions (Mitchell, in press-b). However, such self-pretense does not entail the capacity for planning, because planning arises from the kinesthetic-visual matching abilities required for pretense of another (Mitchell, in press-a, in press-b).

Of course these monkeys may not be *representing* playfighting at all, that is, they may not be using their behavior as a prop in a game of make-believe. Instead, they may have learned that playfighting-like qualities stop other organisms from responding to apparent aggression, such that the combination leads to beneficial results (a level-three interpretation). Still again, such learned activities could be considered self-pretense. Either way, the behavior of these monkeys conflicts with Quiatt's (1984) qualified claim that nonhuman primates are unlikely to use ritualized displays intentionally for manipulation, because they could not psychologically distance themselves enough from these behaviors. If Breuggeman's observations were the only ones showing intentional use of ritualized behaviors, one might question their significance. But some compelling instances of deceptive uses of ritualized behaviors—suggestive of pretense—are also observed in chimpanzees.

Observations of apparently deceptive pretense in normal social relations among chimpanzees (de Waal, 1986; Goodall, 1986) are more frequent than observations of pretend play. De Waal for one provides well-articulated accounts of deception in chimpanzees which can be examined for pretense. In one instance, de Waal tells of a chimpanzee Dandy who (at least once) used a manipulative technique to be able to mate secretly with oestrus females: after noticing something "unusual" outside his enclosure Dandy alarm-barked loudly, attracting the other males in the enclosure to run in the direction of his gaze. Once these males departed, Dandy sexually invited a female. In de Waal's view, the combination of Dandy's actions of initial interest, alarm barking, lack of interest, and immediate sexual solicitation implies intentional deception. However, Dandy is described as noticing something "unusual," and so may simply have taken advantage of the males' departure after his alarm call. Even if the alarm call were intentionally enacted to influence other males to move away, the chimpanzee may not have planned to get rid of the males to copulate with the female. Because he wanted to get near the female, he may have begun to feel anxious around the other males; to relieve his anxiety he acted upon his belief "If I give an alarm call the males will move away," and then found himself (to his delight) alone with the female. At least on the face of it, the chimpanzee need not be described as *pretending* or *feigning* alarm, and he need not have planned to perform the alarm call to be alone with the female.

But then again, he might have. How is one to know? Clearly such individual instances leave much to be desired in terms of evidence, because so many different interpretations are plausible. Many theorists have argued that if we have knowledge of the development of intelligent actions, we would be better able to understand their significance for the organism—how the organism itself interprets its own behavior (Köhler, 1925; Birch, 1945; Mitchell, 1986). Just such a developmental history is supplied (in abbreviated form) by Menzel (1974), who described a series of deceptions by a chimpanzee Belle who tried to thwart a greedy dominant chimp Rock from obtaining hidden food for which Belle knew the location. The development of the deception suggests that Belle tried various means to avoid Rock's finding the food. Belle always led the group of chimps with whom she lived to food when Rock was not present, and her behavior indicated that she intended for the others to follow her to food. However, she approached the food more and more slowly when Rock was present because he took all of it for himself. Belle then avoided uncovering the hidden food if Rock was nearby and sat on the food until he left, but when she retrieved the food Rock learned that she was hiding it and pushed her aside. Next she led the chimps near the food, but stopped before getting to it, which prompted Rock to explore the areas around Belle. Then Belle sat farther from the food and waited until Rock looked away before moving toward it, but Rock apparently began to anticipate Belle's movements and to watch her with his peripheral vision. Sometimes Rock moved away from Belle, but only until she was just about to uncover the food. Rock became highly attentive to any directionality in Belle's movements, searching areas she oriented toward. He also came to recognize that Belle's agitation in relation to his movements suggested that food was nearby. When there were two piles of food, one small and one large, Belle led the group to the smaller pile and then raced for the larger, but this strategy backfired when Rock ignored the smaller pile and attended only to Belle. Belle sometimes even led the group in a direction *opposite* to that of the food, but then quickly ran to the food while Rock searched.

Here we see the development of both Belle's and Rock's knowledge of the social effects of their actions. (Indeed, such psychologically complex interactions seem to support the idea that social knowledge was a significant selective factor in primate evolution—see Whiten & Byrne, 1988.) Available to Belle was the knowledge that Rock moved in the direction of her movements or orientations. Initially, Belle reacted to each of Rock's responses to her actions by suppressing her own behavior and waiting to see what Rock would do before she proceeded. Rock similarly recognized that Belle's behavior was not reliable, and became skeptical, camouflaging his interest in her movements until they became useful. Such actions seem explicable in terms of learning to control and inhibit one's actions.

What needs to be explained is Belle's moving in a direction opposite to the food to get rid of Rock before she approached the food. Clearly Belle had the experience to learn that if she moved in a given direction, Rock searched in that direction. But the leading in the opposite direction is presented as an abrupt change in her strategy. Thus we are in a situation similar to that of Ashley's dog: Belle's leading Rock in a direction opposite to that of the food suggests a plan; she wanted to get rid of Rock so that she could get the food herself. Notice that we cannot appeal to Belle's simply finding herself in a situation which she could exploit, as we did with the Dandy's false alarm calling and Ashley's dog's door-scratching, because Belle's leading away is motiveless outside of a plan, whereas Dandy's alarm call depended upon noticing something "unusual" and Ashley's dog (hypothetically) may have desired to go outside and then changed her mind. That is, circumstances *outside* of those which satisfied the deceptive goal can explain Dandy and the dog, but similar circumstances did not apparently exist for Belle. Thus, Belle's leading Rock away from the food and then running back for it for herself suggest an XYZ plan: if I go in this direction away from the food, he will follow me and search ahead of me, and then when he is searching I can go back and get the food. The fact that Belle also went to the pile of less food first again implicates an XYZ plan: if I lead Rock to the smaller pile, he will take the food there, and I can get the bigger pile for myself. Such plans entail imaginal pretense of some sort (whether or not her leading away from the food can be characterized as *behavioral* pretense), at least when they are first enacted.

Planning seems especially evident in hiding by chimpanzees. When chimpanzees discovered food in the presence of other chimpanzees, they often waited until the others were not around before they retrieved the food. Although such evidence of control in the presence of food can be thought of as learned, in some instances the chimpanzees moved away from the area and only hours later returned to obtain the food (de Waal, 1986; Goodall, 1986). In such instances, an "XY plan" ("I will get the food when others are not around and cannot take it from me") more rudimentary than an XYZ plan can be inferred. The chimp may have learned not to touch the food in the presence of others, but it also *anticipated* returning for the food when others were not around; if others were still around when they returned, presumably the chimp would go away and return later. The hiding present in surreptitious movements in chimps and other animals also implies a plan. For example, both wild chimps and captive gorillas desiring to touch an infant restricted from them will reach behind themselves to touch the infant while facing forward, or will slowly reach out a foot to do so (Goodall, 1986; Mitchell, 1991b). Knowledge of the developmental history of the specific behaviors and their contexts *might* support the claim of a plan, but we lack this knowledge for both chimps and gorillas. Plans of such animals may be mental images of the organism itself participating in to-be-enacted events, but probably exist in less conscious forms. The ability to pretend to enact another's actions implies a kinesthetic-visual matching capacity which creates a fuller representation of the self known through kinesthesis (Mitchell, in press-a, in press-b). Theories that postulate that children or apes come to understand the other by imaginative projection from their own experience (e.g., Gallup, 1985; Harris, 1989) must posit such a translation capacity, yet commonly fail to do so. The translation capacity is necessary to account for the child's recognizing that he or she looks like what the other looks like, because the child cannot see him or herself (see Mitchell, in press-a).

Taking the Perspective of the Other

At the fourth level an organism pretends to itself that its actions or thoughts are literal enactments or experiences of what they represent, or it imagines itself carrying out a series of manipulative enactments. At the fifth level an organism intentionally tries to get another to believe something which the intending organism believes to be false—that is, engage in intentional deception. Instances of nonhuman deception do not fall easily into these two levels (note a similar typological distinction in Lewis, Sullivan, Stanger, & Weiss, 1989; Mitchell, in press-a). Once an animal is capable of planning and pretense, its activities are sufficiently complex to cause observers to question whether or not the animal understands how others interpret its actions. Certainly taking the perspective of the other is evidence of an ability to plan (Mitchell, 1987) because the representational processes involved in the former require the latter (Leslie, 1988). However, the self-consciousness present in planning and pretense, though assisting in the development of a theory of mind of the other, can occur without such perspective-taking (Mitchell, 1990, in press-a, in press-b). Clearly humans take the perspective of the other in innumerable circumstances.

When organisms hide themselves because they do not want another to perceive them, they are hiding at the fifth level. Though apparently obvious from the adult human's perspective, from the human child's perspective such hiding is not a simple operation. Children begin to play hide-and-seek games appropriately when they are about four years of age (Wimmer, Hogrefe, & Sodian, 1988). Prior to that age the understanding of hiding can be egocentric—the child might believe, for example, that by covering her eyes she is effectively "hiding" from the other. One two-year-old friend played hide-and-seek with me by running into another room while my eyes were closed and waiting for me in an open closet! Chimpanzees returning to get hidden food when others are not around suggests perspective-taking, as does their hiding from more dominant chimpanzees (who might interfere with and harm them) when they copulate in areas in which they will remain unseen (de Waal, 1986). A sign-taught pygmy chimpanzee hid objects and himself quite effectively (Savage-Rumbaugh & McDonald, 1988). Antecedents of such hidings should be sought and may influence our interpretation, even though these and other instances of hiding seem to strain credulity at any interpretation other than one requiring the chimpanzee to take the perspective of multiple others. For example, frequently a low-status male used his hand to hide his erect penis from a more dominant male yet allowed it to be seen by a nearby female, all the while surreptitiously looking at the dominant male (de Waal, 1986). Even more than deception, such hiding implicates an animal's taking others' perspectives into account in enacting its intentions. The very commonplace way that observers describe hiding among chimpanzees certainly *suggests* that these organisms know that others can see them. Still, the very same commonplace description pervades depictions of hiding in many nonprimate predators (Mills, 1919; Chauvin & Muckensturm-Chauvin, 1977; McMahan, 1978). The ubiquitousness of hiding in mammals should cause us to be hesitant in our interpretation of hidings—or our interpretation of primate distinctiveness—until we observe and compare the ontogeny of hiding in different species.

In a deception scenario described by de Waal suggestive of both pretense and perspective-taking, a male chimp effected a reconciliation with an adversary by acting as if he noticed something in the grass. Initially, each chimp was aware of the other but neither made a move to reconcile. Then one chimp appeared to find an interesting object, and attracted other chimps (including the adversary) to the spot by loudly hooting. Although the other chimps were quickly disinterested and left, the two adversaries remained excited by the object; in their excitement the two ineluctably touched, and gradually calmed, whereupon one groomed the other. So far the story seems explicable in terms of learning: the calling chimp need only have learned that an alarm call is likely to bring his adversary closer and felt a desire to be with the adversary yet feared approaching him directly. But de Waal adds a captivating gloss to this story: he suggests that the object which so alarmed the caller was nonexistent, in that de Waal himself could never discern the object; and he suggests that the second chimp recognized the deception, perceiving it as an "excuse" to bring the two males together and thus acting as if interested in the object to allow the other chimp to save face. The two chimps engaged in a "collective lie." There is, of course, an alternative explanation which utilizes de Waal's recognition that chimpanzees sometimes hide their embarrassment by attending to something unimportant. Given that the two chimps were former adversaries, it seems likely that these chimps more than the others would be embarrassed or disturbed in their current proximity and so would retain their interest in the "object" as well as their excited state longer than the others.

Even if this explanation is accepted, pretense is still implicated if the chimps attended excitedly to a nonexistent object—in which case they would certainly have feigned interest, as de Waal suggests, in that they were pretending that there was something to be interested in. (Such pretend interest in nothing would argue against the idea of Whiten & Byrne, 1988, that a deceiver must look at a *plausible* object of interest to be effective.) If indeed the chimps did so feign interest, their "collective lie" exhibits both the pretense of the fourth level and the perspective-taking of the fifth level. But we are left with the problem of how to take the apparent "existence" of nothing as representing something. In humans at least, young children require that an object of some kind be physically present if they are to pretend to have an object. The impulse to use *something* to represent another object is so strong that a child given no object from which to pretend to drink searched intently and eventually found a piece of lint to use (Jackowitz & Watson, 1980). Although pretense about objects occurs frequently by 16 months, pretending that nothing represents something occurs infrequently in children even at 23 months. Although in their *play* chimpanzees do not naturally pretend very much about objects (although a pygmy chimpanzee apparently does—see Savage-Rumbaugh & McDonald, 1988), in their *deceptions* chimpanzees (and other primates) appear to pretend a great deal that uninteresting objects are interesting (Bertrand, 1969; de Waal, 1986; Whiten & Byrne, 1988), such that they may gain the requisite experience with self-pretense about objects to be able eventually to represent nothing as something. Thus, Goodall's interpretation of play termite-fishing and solitary aggression as pretend may be accurate, though exactly what is represented by the nothing is unclear.

Some apes, such as the sign-using orangutan Chantek, specify what the nothing represents with signs (Miles, 1986, 1990, personal communication). That is, they use signs as props in a social game of make-believe. Chantek used the signs *cat* and *dog*—animals which frightened and fascinated him—when he wished to prolong or start a walk, acting as though seeking out a hidden cat or dog. At times he also engaged in pretend play about the existence of imaginary cats in which he frightened himself, an activity which began after he evidenced pretense about objects. He also tried to engage his caregivers in pretending that one of the fear-inspiring creatures was outside his trailer window. For example, in one instance he signed *cat* and, with his caregiver in tow, peered out of each of his trailer's windows, but the caregiver could discern no animals.

One can always claim, to discount any evidence of pretense, that actions that look like pretense could result solely from learning, and posit various processes by which primates might have learned to perform these actions. However, it is important to realize that much human pretense could bear the same interpretation, at least when viewed in isolation and from the outside. For example, people sometimes act as if they are about to throw or kick a ball, but then do not, to try to make a dog chase after a nonexistent ball (Mitchell & Thompson, 1991). Such "fakeouts" can be viewed as pretending to throw or kick the ball, but a skeptic might suggest that all one must assume is that the person likes to see the dog move, and knows that when he or she does the incomplete act of "throwing" or "kicking" a ball, the dog runs. Such an analysis is identical to that given for the faked window-slams of the zoo gorilla: just as the gorilla likes to provoke startle *reactions* in people, the person likes to provoke running *reactions* in dogs; neither ape nor human is concerned with influencing the other psychologically. In the case of the person, however, one can ask the person what he or she is doing. And, not surprisingly, the person usually says something like, "I'm trying to get the dog to *think* that I'm throwing the ball," an interpretation that clearly implies pretense. What is intriguing here is that the person interprets his or her actions as attempts to influence the dog mentally. Perhaps with a young child the self-description would be in terms of the dog's behavior, and the original inspiration for the game of fakeout might derive from trial-and-error learning. But by the time one is an adult, one's interpretation of the pretense is in terms of the other's thoughts and beliefs, and the fakeout sequences can become highly variable. This finding suggests that the gorilla who faked window-slams enjoyed her game because she wanted to see if her fakes could *startle* people, not just because she wanted to see if her fakes could make the people *move* in a particular way. One might test this hypothesis by seeing whether or not this gorilla would engage in the fake window-slams with an iconic representation of a person which responded to the window slams, but which was obviously not a person.

Without knowledge of its development, an activity can seem very much like a second-level or third-level activity yet involve planning and taking the perspective of the other. For example, deception in sports can be extremely routinized, such that the deceptions are enacted without conscious thought (Mawby & Mitchell, 1986). But arriving at the point where skill is so effortless requires practice and planning and recognition of how the other will perceive one's actions. Thus, although players do not plan or always take the perspective of the other *explicitly while acting*, these processes are necessary for the creation of the skilled activities in the first place. Just like the person playing fakeout, players in sports describe their actions as directed to influence thinking beings. Thus, thinking thoughts about the other while engaging in a deception is not what is required for fifth-level deception (see Dennett, 1978). What is required is that at some point in the development of the deceptive skill the deceiver take into account how the other would view and respond to the deceiver's actions. In humans, thinking in terms of the other's perspective is so ingrained that even if a deceptive act were developed through trial and error, eventually the person recognizes the other's interpretation of the act. In children, psychological interpretation of the other becomes prevalent and well-formed at about four years of age. At this age the child can mentally represent his or her own perspective as well as another's perspective, and recognize that the two perspectives may differ (DeLoache, 1988). The child comes to understand multiple representations and multiple perspectives of a single reality. If de Waal's interpretations of chimpanzees are correct, at some point the same is true of them. Given that pretense is extremely rare in chimpanzee play but may be rather common in chimpanzee deception (de Waal, 1986), the existence of pretend play in humans may derive evolutionarily from the usefulness of pretense in deception (see, e.g., the various deceptive pretenses described in the Biblical story of David [Frontain, 1990]).

Given our bent toward psychologizing, we should be suspicious of anthropomorphic interpretations of nonhumans. Our psychologizing of others is so ingrained and natural that we approach even obviously nonpsychological phenomena from the same perspective, as in Heider and Simmel's (1944) experiment with moving shapes being perceived as intending to harm, feeling jealous, or being upset. Still, we need to decide whether other organisms also have the same psychologizing tendencies toward one another. Some conclude that they do based on admittedly inadequate evidence (Whiten & Byrne, 1988). Others offer abundant support that, while in some cases equivocal, implies that they do, and suggest experiments that would differentiate distinct psychologies (de Waal, 1986; Gallup, 1985; Miles, 1986). And of course there are always skeptics who deny that it is possible to know how people think about others, let alone how nonhuman animals do. My own tendency is to try to approach the understanding of an animal in terms of (my knowledge of) that animal's past and current experiences, and to see what these experiences would likely lead that organism to believe (assuming that the animal can be affected by these experiences). Such a tendency is commonly used to understand human development in general and our own experience of ourselves, friends, and family in particular, but somehow seems less prevalent in our interpretation of animals.

Taking the Other's Perspective on the Self's Perspective

Once an organism recognizes that the other has a perspective, the organism may come to recognize that that perspective may include the recognition that the organism itself has a perspective. It is at this point that the organism has a self, in the sense that the organism can think about itself from the other's perspective (Dunn, 1988). What kinds of experiences might lead an organism to recognize that the other perceives them psychologically?

Sacks' (1980) analysis of the game Button Button Who's Got the Button suggests that humans commonly have experiences which lead them to recognize the other's perspective on the self's perspective. In this game, the leader appears to place a button in each player's hand, but in fact places it in only one person's hand. The purpose of the game is for the players to guess who has the button. (The game obviously requires more than two players.) In this game, recognizing who has the button is not achieved by seeing the button in that person's hand, but rather by perceiving that the person *knows* that he or she has the button. That is, players experience the others not as exhibiting behaviors, but as *showing their thoughts*. In Button Button, the child learns that she or he can read others' thoughts, but also that others can read her or his thoughts, and that the child can do things to influence the other's interpretation. To devise an effective strategy, the child must develop plans that take into account the other's interpretation of the child's thoughts. The Button Button game offers a means by which children would be led to understand that others are thinking of their mental states. The formal similarity, at least in part, between what happens in the Button Button game and what happened between the chimpanzees Belle and Rock in Menzel's study suggests to me that chimpanzees learn to recognize that the other is construing them as thinking beings. The likelihood that, without language, chimps can move to the even more elaborate knowledge of perspective-taking present in humans is unlikely, but then maybe we do not yet know all there is to know about chimpanzees.

ANIMALS, PRETENSE, AND KNOWLEDGE OF OTHER MINDS

"I am sure she knew, but even after I knew that she knew that I knew that she knew, I still continued to cover up."
—A woman quoted in Werth and Flaherty (1986)

In understanding the mind of another organism, there appear to be two approaches currently in use. In the first approach, associated with Dennett (1978) but reminiscent of Tolman (1949) and others, organisms are viewed as "intentional systems." Characterizing an organism as an intentional system means that we take a stance toward that organism of interpreting its actions as intentional and rational, and remain unconcerned about whether or not the organism is actually intentional and rational, for the sake of the usefulness of this description in explaining and predicting the organism's behavior. In describing, for example, the injury-feigning display of the plover (which seems to me a second-level deception), Dennett writes that the bird intends to give the predator a false belief, making the bird a second-order intentional system (which would seem to be a fifth-level deception according to my analysis). According to Dennett, then, the bird's deception and Belle's deception of Rock by moving in a direction away from the food would be the same psychologically. The other approach, associated with de Waal (1986) but also reminiscent of earlier gestalt, phenomenological, and ethological approaches (see Mitchell, 1986), is to develop a theory about the mental organization of animals of a particular type to understand how these animals perceive and interpret their world. The kind of information obtained by this latter approach provides details about these animals' knowledge at the different levels described in the present framework. We can learn about animals' deficiencies and specializations in perception, learning, pretense, taking the perspective of the other, and so on—in effect, about the knowledge by which they operate. What needs to be added to this approach, I think, is to place the animals' behavior in the developmental context of their own history (Mitchell, 1986, 1987, 1988, 1990).

The approach supported by Dennett seems to prescribe a fourth-level understanding of other creatures. In essense, we engage in pretense about animals' minds, and never concern ourselves with what these animals actually know or understand. In contrast, the approach supported by de Waal offers a fifth-level perspective, in that it invites us to understand the world from their perspective. In so understanding, we may have to justify our interpretations by our own need to experience their behavior as resulting from a coherent set of understandings. Rather than describe animals' behavior in ways that are useful for us without concern for the reality of their experience, I think we should try, as de Waal does, to take their perspective. We may even come to be concerned about their perspective on our perspective—how they interpret us psychologically—a sixth-level analysis. By approaching animals from these higher levels, we gain knowledge about their mental lives, and avoid using them as props in our games of make-believe.

Acknowledgments

I am grateful for suggestions and encouragement from Cathy Hobart, Cathy Clement, Carolyn Saarni, Duane Quiatt, Michael Lewis, and Randy Huff.

References

Alverdez, F. (1927). Täuschung und "Lüge" im Tierreich. In O. Lipmann & P. Plaut (Eds.), *Die lüge in psychologischer, phiosophischer, juristischer, pädagogischer, historischer, soziologischer, sprach- und literaturwissenschaftlicher und entwicklungsgeschichtlicher Betrachtung* (pp. 332–350). Leipzig: Verlag von Johann Ambrosius Barth.

Bateson, G. (1955/1972). A theory of play and fantasy. In *Steps to an ecology of mind* (pp. 177–193). New York: Ballantine Books.

Bertrand, M. (1969). *The behavioural repertoire of the stumptail macaque.* Basel: Karger.

Birch, H. G. (1945). The relation of previous experience to insightful problem solving. *Journal of Comparative Psychology, 38,* 367–383.

Breuggeman, J. A. (1973). Parental care in a group of free-ranging rhesus monkeys (*Macaca mulatta*). *Folia primatologica, 20,* 178–210.

Breuggeman, J. A. (1978). The function of adult play in free-ranging *Macaca mulatta.* In E. O. Smith (Ed.), *Social play in primates* (pp. 169–191). New York: Academic Press.

Chauvin, R., & Muckensturm-Chauvin, B. (1977/1980). *Behavioral complexities*. New York: International Universities Press.

Darwin, C. (1859/1909). *The origin of species*. New York: P. F. Collier & Son.

Darwin, C. (1871/1896). *The descent of man and selection in relation to sex*. New York: D. Appleton & Co.

DeLoache, J. S. (1989). The development of representation in young children. In H. W. Reese (Ed.), *Advances in child development and behavior* (Vol. 22, pp. 1–39). New York: Academic Press.

Dennett, D. C. (1978). *Brainstorms: Philosophical essays on mind and psychology*. Cambridge, MA: Bradford Books.

de Waal, F. (1986). Deception in the natural communication of chimpanzees. In R. W. Mitchell & N. S. Thompson (Eds.), *Deception: Perspectives on human and nonhuman deceit* (pp. 221–244). Albany: SUNY Press.

DiLalla, L. F., & Watson, M. W. (1988). Differentiation of fantasy and reality: Preschoolers' reactions to interruptions in their play. *Developmental Psychology, 24*, 286–291.

Dunn, J. (1988). *The beginnings of social understanding*. Cambridge, MA: Harvard University Press.

Edmunds, M. (1974). *Defence in animals*. Essex, UK: Longman.

Frontain, R.-J. (1990). The trickster tricked: Strategies of deception and survival in the David narrative. In V. L. Tollers & J. Maier (Eds.), *Mappings of the Biblical terrain: The Bible as text* (pp. 170–192). Lewisburg, PA: Bucknell University Press.

Gallup, G. G., Jr. (1985). Do minds exist in species other than our own? *Neurosciences and Biobehavioral Review, 9*, 631–641.

Goodall, J. (1986). *The chimpanzees of Gombe: Patterns of behavior*. Cambridge, MA: Harvard University Press.

Graham, G. (1986). Russell's deceptive desires. *The Philosophical Quarterly, 36*, 223–229.

Groos, K. (1898). *The play of animals*. New York: D. Appleton & Co.

Harris, P. L. (1989). *Children and emotion: The development of psychological understanding*. Oxford, UK: Basil Blackwell.

Heider, F., & Simmel, M. (1944). An experimental study of apparent behavior. *American Journal of Psychology, 57*, 243–259.

Hrdy, S. B. (1979). Care and exploitation of nonhuman primate infants by conspecifics other than the mother. *Advances in the Study of Behavior, 6*, 101–158.

Jackowitz, E. R., & Watson, M. W. (1980). Development of object transformations in early pretend play. *Developmental Psychology, 16*, 543–549.

Köhler, W. (1925/1969). *The mentality of apes*. New York: Liveright Press.

Krebs, J. R. (1977). The significance of song repertoires: The Beau Geste hypothesis. *Animal Behaviour, 25*, 475–478.

Leslie, A. M. (1988). The necessity of illusion: Perception and thought in infancy. In L. Weiskrantz (Ed.), *Thought without language* (pp. 185–210). Oxford, UK: Clarendon Press.

Lewis, M., Sullivan, M., Stanger, C., & Weiss, M. (1989). Self development and self-conscious emotions. *Child Development, 60,* 146–156.

Mason, W. A., & Hollis, J. H. (1962). Communication between young rhesus monkeys. *Animal Behaviour, 10,* 211–221.

Mawby, R., & Mitchell, R. W. (1986). Feints and ruses: An analysis of deception in sports. In R. W. Mitchell & N. S. Thompson (Eds.), *Deception: Perspectives on human and nonhuman deceit* (pp. 313–322). Albany: SUNY Press.

McCune-Nicolich, L. (1981). Toward symbolic functioning: Structure of early pretend games and potential parallels with language. *Child Development, 52,* 785–797.

McMahan, P. (1978). Natural history of the coyote. In R. L. Hall & H. S. Sharp (Eds.), *Wolf and man: Evolution in parallel* (pp. 41–54). New York: Academic Press.

Menzel, E. (1974). A group of young chimpanzees in a one-acre field. In A. M. Schrier & F. Stollnitz (Eds.), *Behavior of nonhuman primates* (Vol. 5, pp. 83–153). New York: Academic Press.

Miles, H. L. (1986). How can I tell a lie? Apes, language, and the problem of deception. In R. W. Mitchell & N. S. Thompson (Eds.), *Deception: Perspectives on human and nonhuman deceit* (pp. 245–266). Albany: SUNY Press.

Miles, H. L. W. (1990). The cognitive foundations for reference in a signing orangutan. In S. T. Parker & K. Gibson (Eds.), *"Language" and intelligence in monkeys and apes: Comparative developmental perspectives* (pp. 511–539). Cambridge, UK: Cambridge University Press.

Mills, E. A. (1919/1976). *The grizzly: Our greatest wild animal.* Sausalito: Comstock Editions.

Mitchell, R. W. (1986). A framework for discussing deception. In R. W. Mitchell & N. S. Thompson (Eds.), *Deception: Perspectives on human and nonhuman deceit* (pp. 3–40). Albany: SUNY Press.

Mitchell, R. W. (1987). A comparative-developmental approach to understanding imitation. In P. P. G. Bateson & P. H. Klopfer (Eds.), *Perspectives in ethology* (Vol. 7, pp. 183–215). New York: Plenum Press.

Mitchell, R. W. (1988). Ontogeny, biography, and evidence for tactical deception. *Behavioral and Brain Sciences, 11,* 259–260.

Mitchell, R. W. (1990). A theory of play. In M. Bekoff & D. Jamieson (Eds.), *Interpretation and explanation in the study of animal behavior, vol. 1: Interpretation, intentionality, and communication* (pp. 197–227). Boulder, CO: Westview Press.

Mitchell, R. W. (1991a). Bateson's concept of "metacommunication" in play. *New Ideas in Psychology, 9,* 73–87.

Mitchell, R.W. (1991b). Deception and hiding in captive lowland gorillas (*Gorilla gorilla gorilla*). *Primates, 32,* 523–527.

Mitchell, R. W. (in press-a). Mental models of mirror-self-recognition: Two theories. *New Ideas in Psychology.*

Mitchell, R. W. (in press-b). The evolution of primate cognition: Simulation, self-knowledge, and knowledge of other minds. In D. Quiatt & J. Itani (Eds.), *Hominid culture in primate perspective*. Denver: University Press of Colorado.

Mitchell, R. W., & Thompson, N. S. (Eds.), (1986). *Deception: Perspectives on human and nonhuman deceit*. Albany: SUNY Press.

Mitchell, R. W., & Thompson, N. S. (1991). Projects, routines, and enticements in dog-human play. In P. P. G. Bateson & P. H. Klopfer (Eds.), *Perspectives in ethology* (Vol. 9, pp. 189–216). New York: Plenum Press.

Morris, M. D. (1986). Large scale deceit: Deception by captive elephants? In R. W. Mitchell & N. S. Thompson (Eds.), *Deception: Perspectives on human and nonhuman deceit* (pp. 183–191). Albany: SUNY Press.

Moynihan, M. (1985). *Communication and noncommunication by cephalopods*. Bloomington, IN: Indiana University Press.

Owen, D. (1980). *Camouflage and mimicry*. Chicago, IL: University of Chicago Press.

Pasteur, G. (1982). A classificatory review of mimicry systems. *Annual Review of Ecology and Systematics, 13*, 169–199.

Piaget, J. (1947/1972). *The psychology of intelligence*. New York: The Free Press.

Quiatt, D. (1984). Devious intentions of monkeys and apes? In R. Harré & V. Reynolds (Eds.), *The meaning of primate signals* (pp. 9–40). Cambridge, UK: Cambridge University Press.

Russow, L.-M. (1986). Deception: A philosophical perspective. In R. W. Mitchell & N. S. Thompson (Eds.), *Deception: Perspectives on human and nonhuman deceit* (pp. 41–51). Albany: SUNY Press.

Saarni, C. (1989). Children's understanding of strategic control of emotional expression in social transactions. In C. Saarni & P. L. Harris (Eds.), *Children's understanding of emotion* (pp. 181–208). Cambridge, UK: Cambridge University Press.

Sacks, H. (1980). Button button who's got the button. *Sociological Inquiry, 50*(3/4), 318–327.

Savage-Rumbaugh, S., & McDonald, K. (1988). Deception and social manipulation in symbol-using apes. In R. Byrne & A. Whiten (Eds.), *Machiavellian intelligence: Social expertise and the evolution of intellect in monkeys, apes, and humans* (pp. 224–237). Oxford: Clarendon Press.

Silverman, P. S. (1986). Can a pigtail macaque learn to manipulate a thief? In R. W. Mitchell & N. S. Thompson (Eds.), *Deception: Perspectives on human and nonhuman deceit* (pp. 151–167). Albany: SUNY Press.

Singer, D. G., & Singer, J. L. (1990). *The house of make-believe: Children's play and the developing imagination*. Cambridge, MA: Harvard University Press.

Tolman, E. C. (1949). *Purposive behavior in animals and men*. Berkeley: University of California Press.

Vander Meer, R. W., & Wojcik, D. P. 1982. Chemical mimicry in the

Myrmecophilous beetle Myrmecaphodius excavaticollis. *Science, 218,* 806–808.

Walton, K. L. (1990). *Mimesis as make-believe: On the foundations of the representational arts.* Cambridge, MA: Harvard University Press.

Werth, L. F., & Flaherty, J. (1986). A phenomenological approach to human deception. In R. W. Mitchell & N. S. Thompson (Eds.), *Deception: Perspectives on human and nonhuman deceit* (pp. 293–311). Albany: SUNY Press.

Whiten, A., & Byrne, R. W. (1988). Tactical deception in primates. *Behavioral and Brain Sciences, 11,* 233–244.

Wickler, W. (1968). *Mimicry in plants and animals.* New York: McGraw-Hill.

Wimmer, H., Hogrefe, J., & Sodian, B. (1988). A second stage in children's conception of mental life: Understanding informational accesses as origins of knowledge and belief. In J. W. Astington, P. L. Harris, & D. R. Olson (Eds.), *Developing theories of mind* (pp. 173–192). New York: Cambridge University Press.

4

The Development of Deception

MICHAEL LEWIS

When we talk about deception, the more polite term for lying, we need to clarify what we mean by the term. Following Bok (1978), it is possible to divide deceptive behavior into three large categories. While not totally inclusive of all cases of deception, these three categories capture a good deal of what we usually refer to when we speak of deception: Deceptive behavior can take the form of lying to save the feelings of another, lying to avoid punishment, and lying to the self. Each of these forms of deception makes its appearance, in the life of a child, at young ages. In order for us to understand its developmental course, as well as differences between individuals and groups, we need to distinguish between these different forms.

LYING TO PROTECT THE FEELINGS OF ANOTHER

Felicia is a three-year-old girl who is eagerly awaiting a Christmas present from her grandmother. She is hoping for an attractive toy. The day after Christmas, her grandmother presents her with a knitted sweater. Felicia rips open the package, sees the sweater and smiles at her grandmother. Turning to her, she says, "I'm going to wear it right now."

Felicia, like many children of her age, has already learned how to deceive. She has masked her facial expression. Instead of showing disappointment and sadness, she smiles. She announces how much she enjoys the gift. Felicia has learned the social rule pertaining to deception in the service of protecting another's feelings. Many examples like this can be found, and they apply to adults as well as children.

Consider the situation where you are invited to a dinner party and are served an absolutely terrible meal. At the end of the dinner, your host and hostess thank you for coming and ask you if you enjoyed the meal. Instead of responding with a truthful statement like, "It was an inedible meal," we are likely to respond with some nicety such as, "It was delicious."

We do this in order to save the feelings of the other. Examples of this type of behavior suggest that this form of deception is useful in that it allows us to maintain social commerce, and allows us to compliment one another, even in the face of events that could be interpersonally painful. One might argue that the function of deception in protecting the feelings of others is evolutionarily appropriate if one of the tasks of our evolutionary history was to develop and maintain complex social interactions. Although some might say that such deception is destructive to interpersonal relationships, it does seem reasonable to assume that the maintenance of social interactions requires deceptions of this kind.

Perhaps an example of such interpersonal necessity can be seen in this example: A wife comes home from a shopping day and shows her husband a dress that she had bought on sale. She exclaims how much she loves this dress and how well it looks on her. Moreover, she informs her husband that, because it was a sale, she has saved money; however, she cannot return it to the store. It would seem appropriate under such circumstances for her husband to tell her how he likes her choice in spite of the fact that he finds it unattractive. He does so because it allows him to preserve the good feelings of his wife and, at the same time, allows him to feel good about himself for being able to give his wife pleasure in spite of the fact that he does not like it. It other words, deception of this type has significant altruistic signifi-cance and should be considered in this regard. Of course, the task is to deceive in such a way as to lead the other to believe what you do or say is what you really think or feel. It would achieve nothing to deceive and have the person detect the deception. Thus, the task of individuals who seek to deceive in order to preserve the feelings of others must be to make sure that their deception is successful.

Children learn the rule about such deceptive practices from significant others, most often from their parents or older siblings. They learn to protect the feelings of others through both direct instruction as well as indirect observation of parental behavior. Consider, for example, the direct teaching as exemplified by the case of grand-mother's sweater. Children are instructed by their parents to deceive in order to protect the feelings of another. They are told, "Tell grandmother you like the sweater even though you were hoping for a toy"; that is, they are led to believe that there are occasions when deception is appropriate. They are also informed about deception indirectly. In such cases, children observe that their parents engage in deception to save the feelings of others, even though the children are not direct participants in these exchanges. This indirect learning is an important feature of early socialization (Lewis & Feiring, 1981). Consider the following example that was relayed to me by a parent of one of our subjects. Rhoda, the mother, reported the following incident: Several weeks earlier, she had been expecting a visit from her friend, who was coming to the house to have coffee. Prior to her friend's arrival, Rhoda discovered that she had many things that she needed to do and was unhappy that her time would be taken up with her friend's visit. She exclaimed, in the presence of her child, "I have so much to do. I really wish she wouldn't come." Almost immediately after stating this desire, Sally's mother rang the doorbell and appeared in the doorway, at which point Rhoda exclaimed, again in the presence of her child, how glad she was to see her.

Here, we see how indirect teaching of deceptive behavior can take place with young children. Both directly and indirectly, children are taught by their parents to deceive in order to spare the feelings of another. I suspect that deception is also taught indirectly when parents make clear to their children the moral importance of sparing the feelings of another, and when they teach altruistic and empathic behavior. The child is likely to learn early in life that there is competition between truthfulness and sparing the feelings of others, and may decide to order these two moral dilemmas in favor of the lie.

There are few studies that explore directly this form of deception—one exception is the work of Saarni (1984). In this experiment children are promised an attractive toy if they satisfy a task requirement. After having done so, they are then presented with a less attractive toy and their facial expressions are observed. This direct observation of children's ability to use deception, in a lifelike situation, was not a test of the use of lying to protect the feelings of others, although it might be assumed that the children's masking their facial expression was an attempt to protect the feelings of the experimenter by not showing disappointment over the toy reward. First-, third-, and fifth-graders were placed in a situation where their expectations for the desirable toy were not met. With increasing age, children demonstrated increased ability to mask their internal states, with girls showing this ability earlier, and to a greater extent than boys.

More recently, Saarni (personal communication, 1991) attempted to manipulate children's feelings about the experimenter in order to see if she could elicit sympathy toward the experimenter and, therefore, greater masking of the children's emotional behavior. Only limited support was found for the hypothesis that children will mask negative behavior in order to spare the feelings of another. Unfortunately, other than clinical observation, this form of deception has received little attention.

LYING TO AVOID PUNISHMENT

The most common form of lying, at least in early childhood, has to do with deception around transgressions likely to result in punishment. Children soon learn to lie when they are asked by adults whether or not they have committed a transgression. So, for example, a two-year-old child is told not to eat a cookie, but, when the mother is no longer present, the child proceeds to eat it. Later, when the mother questions the child about eating the cookie, the child admits that she* has done so. Upon hearing that the child has not been obedient, the parent becomes angry or upset and punishes the child. Children are not stupid, nor are they foolish. After only one or two interactions like this, the child discovers that if she admits to eating the cookie, she will be punished. She lies to avoid the punishment.

Around events which are easily detectable, parents discover that their children are lying. A new socialization rule is established to meet the child's behavior. The strategy the parent next adopts is to inform the child that: (1) it is "bad" to lie, and (2) the child will be punished if he tells a lie. Now the child is confronted with a more difficult problem. If he tells the truth about his transgression, he will be punished. If he lies, he will be punished. It does not take very long for the child to learn that for many categories of transgression and of lying, it is impossible for the parent to tell whether or not the transgression has taken place. When this discovery is made, the child lies with the hopes of avoiding punishment.

In one family in our studies there were two children, a girl of 3+ and a boy of 2, who, when confronted with the fact that a transgression had been committed, at least by one of them, decided to lie and tell the mother that they had not done it. The mother, knowing full well that one of them was responsible, presented them with another moral dilemma. Not knowing which one was the culprit, she declared, "If

---

*"She" and "he" will be used randomly when referring to children. This allows me to avoid the plural form (children) or the s/he, his/her form.

you don't tell me which one of you did it, then I will punish both of you. The child who did it will be responsible for an innocent child being blamed and punished." Such moral dilemmas are often pointed out to children. If, indeed, a mother maintains her position and punishes both of them, they soon learn that: (1) they will not be found out, (2) it is not good to "rat on the other," and (3) she is likely to punish both of them less severely than she would the one who actually transgressed. As we can see, children are confronted with the issue of deception to avoid punishment at quite an early age.

Although there are many studies of children's ability to deceive and of children's understanding of deception, there are few studies that actually explore children's behavior when they violate a transgression (see DePaulo, Stone, & Lassiter, 1985; DePaulo, Jordan, Irvine, & Laser, 1982; Feldman, Jenkins, & Popoola, 1979, for some studies on older children's ability to deceive). One can choose to study what it is that children know about deception, that is, their ideas and cognition in regard to deception and in regard to lying to avoid punishment, and/or one can study what they actually do. I do not believe that there is necessarily a strong correspondence between their actions and their understanding of their actions, a distinction pointed out by others in terms of the development of functions and ability (see Piaget, 1965).

There are many problems in the study of deception, some of which have to do with children's understanding. For example, young children can be asked to pretend to deceive (Feldman & White, 1980). In one study, they were given a drink that was slightly sour and told to pretend that they liked it, or, alternatively, they were asked to pretend that they were having an emotional experience, such as being sad, happy, or surprised, when they were not. Both instances require not only the ability to deceive, but also the ability to play act. Moreover, they require that the child understand the adult experimenters' instruction in regard to what it is they want them to do. Such factors as these are likely to be related to the child's language understanding and to other more complex cognition skills such as intentional pretending. What such paradigms do not do is to get at the actual behavior of children in particular situations; for example, situations in which they have been asked not to do something, then violate the prescription, and then have to choose whether or not to lie about their action. In such a paradigm, one is able to observe very young children's behavior, independent of the child's verbal ability to understand the elaborate instructions of what it is the adult wants the child to do and independent of the elaborate cognitive abilities which are necessitated by pretending to deceive.

In the particular set of studies that my colleagues and I carried out, we employed a very simple paradigm (Lewis et al., 1989, in press). The results, which I summarize here, are based upon it. The child is brought into a room where, unknown to the child, the child is videotaped. While the child is sitting at a table, the experimenter, behind the child, unpacks and constructs an elaborate and complex toy. While doing so, the experimenter instructs the child not to turn around and look at the toy that is being set up. The experimenter encourages the child not to look and informs the child that the child will be able to look and play with the toy some time later. After the toy is constructed, the experimenter informs the child that she must leave the room for a few minutes. The experimenter tells the child not to look at the toy while she is gone. The experimenter leaves and the child is left in the room for 5 minutes if he does not look at the toy, or until he turns around and looks. As soon as the child looks, the experimenter returns to the room and looks at the child. This is called the *stare condition*, which lasts for 5 to 10 seconds. Immediately afterward, in the *question condition*, the experimenter says to the child, "Did you peek?" The child's verbal response, as well as its facial and bodily behavior, are recorded and scored from the videotapes.

This simple paradigm allows us to observe what children would do in a real life situation in which they have violated a rule that some adult has asked them to conform to. While this may be a prototype for the general proposition of deceiving in order to avoid punishment, it must be mentioned that the violated act does not constitute a serious moral violation (but then, again, neither does eating a cookie, nor not doing one's homework, nor not washing behind one's ears). Moreover, the child does not know, nor is she told, the nature of the punishment or whether punishment will occur if she violates the prohibition. Both of these variables constitute important aspects of the problem which need further elaboration. Even so, such a paradigm does have the advantage of a real-life quality, does not necessitate pretend deception, and can be used with very young children because of its limited verbal complexity.

DECEPTION IN THE VERY YOUNG

In a series of studies, my colleagues and I have examined age, sex, and cultural differences in deceptive behavior. We have also considered whether or not children's intellectual ability is related to their deception. Finally, we determined whether or not children's lying is detectable.

In the first study, with Catherine Stanger and Margaret Sullivan, we looked at deception in children not quite 3 years old (Lewis, Stanger, & Sullivan, 1989). There were three major findings. First, we found that the majority of the subjects peeked when left alone. Only four or approximately 10% of the children did not look. Of the subjects who looked, 38% told the truth and said they did look. Thirty-eight percent lied and said they did not look. Twenty-four percent gave no verbal response to the question. Thus, only 38% of the children were willing to admit to a transgression that they had just performed. Second, interesting differences related to sex were noted. Although there were too few subjects who did not peek, 75% of those who resisted looking were girls. However, of the children who peeked, boys were more likely than girls to admit to the transgression. Of the children who denied peeking or did not respond, the great majority were girls, whereas of those who admitted their transgression, the majority were boys. Third, through the use of an elaborate coding system that measured both facial as well as bodily postures, we found that we could not distinguish between those children who did not lie and those that did. Such findings as these indicate that children under three years of age are already capable of lying when they violate a rule.

Age and Sex Differences in Lying

In the next series of studies, my colleagues, Margaret Sullivan, Kiyoko Kawakami, and Kiyobumi Kawakami, and I observed children between the ages of 3+ and 6 years of age. Figure 1 presents the percentage of children saying, "Yes"; that is, they admitted that they looked. It is important to note that above 3 years of age, the great majority of children lied when asked if they peeked. Although no sex differences were found in children's deceptive behavior, the girls were significantly less likely to peek than the boys (see Figure 2). This finding is consistent with our earlier result and indicates that girls resist temptation better than boys. As might be expected, as children become older, they become better at resisting temptation (Mischel & Ebbesen, 1970). In this task, resisting temptation means that the child sat for five minutes with nothing to do and did not look at the toy. Even so, by 6 years of age, 35% of the children were able to do this.

Lying and IQ

We next sought to determine the relation between children's IQ and their likelihood of lying. Although at first it appears to be counter-intuitive, there is good reason to believe that lying in order

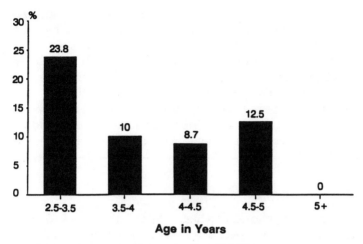

Figure 1. Percentage of children saying "Yes" by age.

not to be punished is an adaptive response. As such, one might expect to find that children who are better able to mask their true feelings and who do not confess might have a higher IQ than those who do. Indeed, there is evidence to indicate that successful masking of emotion and deception is associated with general social skills and is related to adjustment (Wheldall & Alexander, 1985).

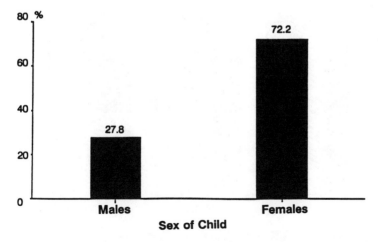

Figure 2. Percentage of children not peeking by sex.

In order to assess the relation between deception and IQ, the Peabody Picture Vocabulary Task, a measure of verbal IQ, was administered to children who also received the deception test. Figure 3 presents IQ scores as a function of whether or not the children lied. Significant IQ differences were found: for both boys and girls, children who admitted their transgression showed significantly lower IQs than those who lied or did not peek. The difference between those who lied and those who did not peek was not significant. Thus, children who told the truth and did not lie when questioned about their peeking had the lowest IQs.

Facial/Bodily Masking While Lying

For those children who lied when asked if they peeked, the next question we wanted to answer was how successful those children were in masking their facial and bodily behavior. We explored the children's ability to deceive in two ways. In the first, we coded the facial and bodily behavior of the children as they were stared at and when they answered the question, "Did you peek?" Some of the behaviors scored were the presence of a relaxed face, smiling, frowning, nervous touching, biting of the lips, and gaze aversion. We wanted to determine if these and other facial and bodily behaviors were different for the children who lied or told the truth. The second way in which we explored this problem of masking was to edit the

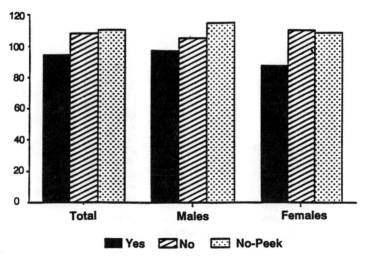

Figure 3. Mean IQ of response group by sex.

videotapes and produce vignettes of the child's answer to the question. These vignettes were shown to adults varying in age, sex, and experience as parents. Only two types of children's response were shown in the vignettes: those children who said "No" and did not peek, and those children who said "No" but did peek.

The results from both types of analyses were remarkably similar. Neither the detailed analysis of facial and bodily behavior coded by experimenters trained in facial coding procedure, nor the overall estimates by adults varying in age, sex, and experience with children, showed that these different groups of children could be differentiated. The careful coding system revealed no differences between truth tellers, liars, and non-peekers. Moreover, there were no differences in the adult's ability, beyond chance level, in detecting non-peekers from liars. This latter finding was true as a function of age and sex of the children being observed, as well as the age, sex, and experience of the adult observers. The results indicate that in this simple task of deception, children from 3+ to 6 years of age are able to deceive adults without being detected.

Having found that children, as a group, are able to deceive, it was important to observe individual differences. There were some children who were terrible at deception, who were readily differentiated from other children who deceived and could not be detected. Some children appeared to be excellent deceivers, that is, few observers reported that when they said, "No, I did not look," they were lying. Where these individual differences originate and whether or not they are characteristics that will be maintained over childhood remains to be seen. What is clear is that, certainly among adults, there are vast differences in deceptive ability. Whether these individual differences in childhood remain consistent over the life span is unknown, but may exist by three years of age.

Cultural Differences

In order to determine whether or not this paradigm would suit a different culture, and in order to determine whether or not similar findings would be obtained if the study were performed elsewhere, Japanese children between the ages of four and seven were presented with the same paradigm. This study was carried out in Tokyo. Although there was not a complete overlap in ages between the American and Japanese samples, consistent findings were found. First, the paradigm appeared to be successful as a method of exploring deception among Japanese children. Second, like Americans, Japanese children, as they become older, are more likely to deceive. No differences were found between American and Japanese children in this regard. Perhaps most interestingly, Japanese children were more likely than American children to resist temptation; that is, among comparable age children, proportionally more Japanese children were able to go five minutes without peeking than were their American counterparts. Observation of the facial and bodily behavior of the Japanese children who lied, as compared to those who did not or who did not peek, also revealed the children's ability to successfully deceive. No differences between groups were found using the facial/bodily coding systems described for the American sample. One cultural difference did emerge which is consistent with the differences reported between Japanese and Americans. Although patterns were similar for children of both cultures, Japanese children showed less facial behavior, less smiling, lip biting, frowning, and nervous touching, than did American children (see Lewis, 1989).

THE MEANING OF DECEPTION

Taken together, these findings on children's ability to deceive indicate that deception, in order to avoid punishment, is a skill learned early in life. Moreover, children's deception increases over the first six years of life. Children with higher IQs are more likely to deceive than children with lower IQs. Studies which report changes in ability as a function of age and as a function of IQ usually refer to skills that are advantageous for the child. In this case, however, we see that children, as they get older, lie more and become better liars. Moreover, children with higher IQs are better able to lie. Given our belief in the moral reprehensibility of lying, why should it be the case that children improved in their lying skills and learned to lie so well, so young? I would suggest that the answer to this puzzle lies in the functional use of lying in this type of situation.

Lying to avoid punishment, I believe, should be considered as part of a general scheme related to self-preservation. People lie in order to avoid injury to the self that would result from admitting they violated a transgression. This does not mean that, from a moral point of view, we should view lying as acceptable behavior. Rather, it may mean that lying may be considered to be "natural action" in the service of adaptation and survival. The predicament that such a finding presents can be seen when we confront parents' concern for their children's lying.

I am often asked by parents what they should do when they discover that their child has lied. Take, for example, the case of Sally who has gone to her friend Ruth's house and brings home Ruth's toy which she claims was given to her. Sally's mother accepts Sally's story of the gift, until she receives a phone call from Ruth's mother who tells her that Sally has taken the toy and asks if she would return it. Sally has lied to her mother and her mother is angry at Sally for being lied to. She says, "Don't lie to me!" What is to be noticed is that Sally's mother focuses on the lie rather than on the child's stealing of the toy. Our analysis of situations like this reveals that parental upset over their children's lying and their focus on the child's lie is predicated on their belief that the child's lie reflects a breakdown in the interpersonal relationship between parent and child. It goes something like, "Sally should not lie to me. She does not have a good relationship with me if she lies." If our results are meaningful, what Sally's behavior indicates is not so much a breakdown in her interpersonal relationship with her mother as it is her "natural desire" to avoid punishment. This act of self-preservation does not reflect a failure in her interpersonal relationship with her mother. Perhaps more important, her mother, by focusing on her child's lie, has neglected the more important moral issue of Sally's stealing.

In discussions with parents, I have tried to point out that lying may be a reasonable strategy to avoid punishment. We cannot expect our children not to lie in order for them to maintain their need for self-preservation. What we need to do as parents and educators is to focus the child on the transgression itself rather than on the act of lying. Sally should be taught and made to focus on her stealing of Ruth's toy. If she learns not to steal, then she will not need to lie.*

This need for self-preservation appears to be a powerful one, one to which most of us are committed. When I have presented the moral dilemma in a slightly different fashion, it becomes quite clear to adults that lying for self-preservation is an action, in some circumstances, which they would be likely to do. For example, if we lived in a culture in which the stealing of an apple would result in the chopping off of a hand as punishment for the transgression, and if we were asked did we steal the apple, few among us would admit to the transgression. It seems more than reasonable that we would lie in order to preserve our hand. Thus, lying for self-preservation is an action that many of us would undertake, especially if the punishment was as draconian as losing a hand. There might be a relation between severity of

---

*I would hope that children would not lie; however, the data from at least two cultures indicate that this is not so. Lying is not morally correct, however 'natural' it might be. Nevertheless, it appears that few children and adults will avoid lying if it means self-protection from punishment.

punishment and lying behavior. In order to explore whether severe punishment by parents was more or less likely to be associated with children's lying when they committed a transgression, we obtained a measure of parental punishment style and compared it to children's truth telling or lying behavior in the peek situation. In general, we found an association between more severe punishment and a greater incidence of lying. Although the causal nature of this association has not been firmly determined, it seems reasonable, at least as a working assumption, to postulate that severe parental punishment for transgression is more likely, rather than less likely, to contribute to lying and deceptive behavior. Thus, lying and self-preservation appear to be related.

SELF-DECEPTION

The third general class of deception or lying is probably the most frequent; lying to the self or self-deception. Self-deception, like the other forms of deception, has both positive and negative features. For example, when an adult female refuses to believe that the lump she feels in her breast could possibly be cancer, she is deceiving herself into thinking that this is a benign fibrous growth; then she is likely to suffer serious consequences including death for her self-deception. On the other hand, it is often advantageous for the maintenance of self-esteem to deceive oneself in order to continue to act in the world. For example, a college student patient of mine reported to me that he had asked a girl out on a date on three occasions, and on all three occasions she had been busy and unable to go out with him. He concluded that he was not interested in dating such a person because he did not want to compete with so many other people for her attention. He did not wish to consider the possibility that his repeated requests for a date, meeting with no success, was a marker of her indifference to him and her desire not to go out on a date with him.

In this case, the young man was able to preserve his self-esteem in the face of this apparent rejection and thus was able to ask others out for a date where he could be more successful. In like fashion, it has been reported that some patients, when told they are terminally ill, are likely to fall apart and be completely incapacitated by their reactions, whereas others deny their illnesses and continue to put their lives in order (Miller & Green, 1985). Self-deception has been explored by others and constitutes a rich literature (see, for example, Chapter 2, this volume).

While self-deception is an area of considerable interest in adult behavior, there is almost no literature on self-deception in children, nor are there any theories about its development. Any theory about the development of self-deception requires that the organism be capable of self-reflection and, at the same time, capable of denying the product of the self-reflection. We know, of course, from a variety of sources that children, by the age of two to three years, are capable of self reflection and are capable of evaluating their own behavior, vis-à-vis standards, values, and goals of others as well as themselves (see Lewis, 1992). How this capacity interacts with self-deception remains a topic to be further explored.

THE LIES OF CHILDREN

Most of the research on deception involves older children, their ability to deceive, the antecedents of that ability, and the meaning of deception for a theory of mind. I have chosen not to deal with these areas because it would take us far afield from the topic at hand. It does appear obvious that in order for a child to deceive, the child must know: (1) what is expected, (2) compare what is expected to what he has done, (3) consider the consequence of the violation, and (4) know what behaviors are likely to be successful in "fooling" the other into thinking he is not deceiving or lying. This, of course, implies that the child has knowledge of himself, knowledge of his own mind, knowledge of the other's mind, and knowledge that the other has knowledge of his mind. This recursive pattern of knowing of others and oneself forms the basis for a theory of mind (see, for example, Chandler, Fritz, & Hala, 1989; Godian, 1989).

In our work, we have been less interested in the cognitive underpinnings of deception and more interested in children's real life ability to mask their emotions. Moreover, we have focused upon what the child does, not what the child thinks or the child's explanation of what she has done. It is clear from observations that children are capable of deception in both their verbal behavior as well as masking their facial and bodily behavior. One might argue, however, that adult human forms of deception can only be said to have occurred if one can prove that the child knows what was expected and intentionally deceives the observer. Without such proof of intention, the evidence for which can only be obtained through questioning the child's knowledge, we do not really know whether cognitive-based deception has taken place. While I appreciate the form that the argument takes, it seems to me that observations other than direct questioning can reveal to us children's intentional behavior (see Lewis, 1990). For example, we can observe children's facial and bodily expression in the peek situation when they are left alone in the room, both before and after they actually look at the toy, and compare it to what they look like when the experimenter enters the room. We have found that children's facial expressions, as they violate the prohibition, show much more concern and disturbance than the face they assume when the experimenter enters the room. In other words, children alter their facial expression as a consequence of the appearance of the adult. While this type of evidence can never substitute for a verbal report of "I deliberately altered my face so as to fool the experimenter," they do constitute sufficient evidence to allow us to conclude that the child is actively engaging in deception. If this is the case, then it is quite clear that the three forms of deception that we have mentioned are likely to be learned early and used by children in order to negotiate the complex and multifaceted social world in which they live and on which they are dependent.

References

Bok, S. (1978). *Lying: Moral choice in public and private life*. New York: Vintage Books.

Chandler, M., Fritz, A. S., & Hala, S. (1989). Small-scale deceit: Deception as a marker of two-, three-, and four-year-olds' early theories of mind. *Child Development, 60*, 1263–1277.

DePaulo, B. M., Jordan, A., Irvine, A., & Laser, P. S. (1982). Age changes in the detection of deception. *Child Development, 53*, 701–709.

DePaulo, B. M., Stone, J. I., & Lassiter, G. D. (1985). In R. Schlenker (Ed.), *The self and social life* (pp. 323–370). New York: McGraw-Hill.

Godian, B. (1989). *The development of deception in young children.* Paper presented at SRCD Meeting, Kansas City, Missouri.

Feldman, R., Jenkins, L., & Popoola, O. (1979). Detection of deception in adults and children via facial expression. *Child Development, 50,* 350–355.

Feldman, R., & White, J. (1980). Detecting deception in children. *Journal of Communication, 30,* 121–129.

Lewis, M. (1989). Culture and biology: The role of temperament. In P. Zelazo & R. Barr (Eds.), *Challenges to developmental paradigms* (pp. 203–226). Hillsdale, NJ: Lawrence Erlbaum Associates.

Lewis, M. (1990). The development of intentionality and the role of consciousness. *Psychological Inquiry, 1*(3), 231–248.

Lewis, M. (1992). *Shame, the exposed self.* New York: The Free Press.

Lewis, M., & Feiring, C. (1981). Direct and indirect interactions in social relationships. In L. Lipsitt (Ed.), *Advances in infancy research* (Vol. 1, pp. 129–161). Norwood, NJ: Ablex.

Lewis, M., Stanger, C., & Sullivan, M. (1989). Deception in three-year-olds. *Developmental Psychology, 25*(3), 439–443.

Lewis, M., Sullivan, M., Kawakami, K., & Kawakami, K. (in press). Studies in deception: Age, sex, IQ, and cultural differences.

Miller, S. M., & Green, M. I. (1985). Coping with stress and frustration: Origins, nature and development. In M. Lewis & C. Saarni (Eds.), *The socialization of emotion* (pp. 263–314). New York: Plenum.

Mischel, W., & Ebbesen, E. B. (1970). Attention in delay of gratification. *Journal of Personality and Social Psychology, 26,* 329–337.

Piaget, J. (1965). *The moral judgment of the child.* New York: The Free Press.

Saarni, C. (1984). An observational study of children's attempts to monitor their expressive behavior. *Child Development, 55,* 1504–1513.

Wheldall, K., & Alexander, R. (1985). The deception study: A related paradigm for the evaluation of generalizability of social skill training. *Behavioral Psychology, 13,* 342–348.

5

The Socialization of Emotional Dissemblance

CAROLYN SAARNI
MARIA VON SALISCH

PAUL (6 years): You don't want to show them that it hurts, because then they'll think you're a cry-baby.

CYNTHIA (9 years): When she just ignored me and invited the other girls instead to her party, I didn't show my hurt. I said to all of them that she was stupid anyway, and I wouldn't want to go to her stupid old party.

JARED (11 years): Well, it depends on whom you're with. Like I'd show how I feel to my friend Nick, but even with him I sometimes can't show or tell him my opinion because it might hurt his feelings.

JULIA (14 years): I used to think that I couldn't show my feelings to people unless they were my best friends or my parents, you know, only people I could trust. But now it matters to me how I feel; if the feeling is important or is about something important, then I'm going to show it, and that's just too bad if someone doesn't like it.

The preceding interview responses from children capture the richness of how children come to make sense of the fact that in our culture (and Western cultures more generally) we teach children a contradiction in values: "You should be honest," and at the same time, "your genuine ("honest") feelings may have to be expressed deceptively." There is a labyrinthine set of rules and expectations regarding what to express emotionally, where, when, and to whom. Impressively enough, by middle childhood children have learned or constructed for themselves an implicit set or rules and contingencies for figuring out under what conditions which emotions may be expressed and to whom. From our perspective, this growth in complexity of emotional expression is inseparable from the sorts of relationships children have. Thus, for example, children growing up in homes with alcoholic parents or who are abused seem to operate with a somewhat different set of rules about how and with whom to express their feelings than do children who grow up in more functional families. These rules reveal themselves most clearly as expectations that people hold about whether to express how one feels straightforwardly and genuinely, indirectly, or deceptively. When we show our feelings indirectly or deceptively in our faces, in our tone of voice, and in our body movement, we are *dissembling* our emotional communication to others. Just as the children's comments at the beginning of this essay showed, dissemblance of feelings is very much related to whom we are with and to what we are really feeling.

What we shall present in this chapter are recent research findings and theories about how children acquire strategies of dissemblance for emotional expression and communication. We shall include a discussion of how cognitive development is relevant to emotional dissemblance; what motivates children to dissemble will also be considered. After describing how social competence and emotion management are linked, we shall also address adaptive versus maladaptive emotional dissemblance.

STRATEGIES OF DISSEMBLANCE

When we alter our external expression of our feelings, we often are attempting to bring our expressive behavior into accordance with our beliefs about what is appropriate or socially desirable under certain circumstances. These beliefs about what expressions of emotions are socially desirable or appropriate are referred to as *display rules*. The term "display" refers to what we see in someone's facial expression, and the use of the word "rule" means that there is considerable social consensus or predictability about what sort of facial expression is displayed. Ekman and Friesen (1975) introduced four prototypical strategies for characterizing how adults in our culture may modify their emotional behavior when they attempt to put display rules into practice. These display rule strategies include *minimization*, which is tantamount to miniaturizing the display of one's genuine feelings (e.g., you are really quite angry, but your expression looks more like irritation: perhaps you knit your brow and press your lips together tightly); *maximization*, which is an exaggerated expression of how one really feels (e.g., you wake up feeling tired, but you adopt an expression of pain and distress as you tell your spouse that you just have to sleep-in

that morning); *masking,* which is adopting a neutral expression or
"poker face" (e.g., you are alone on a subway car and two
menacing-looking young adults get on; you mask your feeling of
apprehension with a blank, neutral expression); and *substitution,*
which entails expressing an emotion that is altogether different from
what one actually feels (e.g., you feel anxious, but you present a smile
to your audience). These expressive strategies have been observed in
children, and although their order of emergence does not appear to be
fixed, we speculate that minimization and maximization appear first in
children's expressive strategy repertoires. Figuring out a substitution or
how to put on a poker-face may require somewhat more complexity of
thought and greater command of facial musculature, and we would
assume that children will demonstrate these expressive strategies
somewhat later. However, what is astonishing is that minimization
and maximization may already be occurring in the second year of life
and perhaps even earlier (e.g., a toddler might cry when his older
sibling teases him in order to dramatize his apparent distress for the
purpose of bringing a parent to his aid) . What this suggests is that
human beings are remarkably responsive to social influence when it
comes to modification of their emotional–expressive behavior. An
additional important implication is that early in life emotional–
expressive behavior is also subject to self-control or volition, *to some
degree.* (As we shall discuss below, high emotional intensity is
identified by children as the primary reason when emotions are
genuinely expressed, often because very intense emotions are not felt
as though they are controllable.)

Evidence for toddlers acquiring the display rule strategies of
minimization and maximization is indirect. Malatesta and Haviland
(1982), who observed infants in the first year of life, found that
mothers tended to attend to their babies' negative emotional behavior
less often as the infants got older. The infants also began to reduce
their intensity of negative emotional displays as they got older.
Malatesta and Haviland inferred that mothers were socializing their
young infants to minimize expressions of negative emotion. On the
other hand, considerable anecdotal evidence is available from parents
and pediatricians alike that, toward the end of the first year, infants
will exaggerate their distress if they determine that a parent is nearby
and that they can get their attention with this strategy; when alone or
not in the company of a parent, their distress may appear to be more
inhibited. By the time we get to young preschoolers, observational
research does exist that provides more direct evidence for children
minimizing and maximizing the expressive display of their emotions.
For example, the ethologist Blurton-Jones observed young children in

a playground accidentally injuring themselves in a minor way; if the mother was not in the vicinity or did not look at them, the child went on playing. However, if the mother looked at the child or was close by, then the child let out a shriek and moaned over an ostensible injury (Blurton-Jones, 1967). What we see in these observations, whether systematic or anecdotal, is that young children use their emotional–expressive behavior to control social consequences for themselves. We will return to this topic as part of our discussion of motives and reinforcers for emotional dissemblance.

Cultural and Personal Display Rules

Display rules can take a couple of different forms. The first is *cultural* display rules: These take the form of social conventions or norms that prescribe how one should express one's feelings, even if one does not feel the emotion that would correspond to the acceptable facial expression. For example, one would not normally show one's displeasure at receiving an unwanted gift if the gift-giver expects one to like it. Cultural display rules have the added advantage in that they are generally agreed to by most members of a culture or subculture, and thus they permit smooth, predictable social exchange. For example, imagine yourself in a clothing shop. You try on a couple of jackets but in the end decide not to buy anything in the store. You politely thank the salesperson for his help, and instead of smiling back (perhaps even a bit peremptorily), he bursts into tears. Suddenly you are catapulted into an *un*predicted and *personal* social transaction with him as opposed to the more customary and predictable exchange between customer and salesperson. In this example we also deliberately used the male gender for the salesperson so that cultural display rules surrounding men's crying would also be illustrated (i.e., they generally "should not" cry, or at least not in impersonal situations).

Personal display rules are often more idiosyncratic, and their function differs from cultural display rules as well. Whereas the latter is for the sake of predictable and conventional social exchanges, personal display rules function to help one feel as though one is coping more adequately with an emotionally taxing situation. For example, 11-year-old Ruth experienced what she presumed was a painful rejection by a close friend. When the friend was encountered again, Ruth adopted emotional–expressive behavior that was a cool, impervious, supremely self-confident exterior. Inside she felt anger and sadness but did not reveal them to her friend. Ruth felt that she needed to protect her vulnerability at having been rejected, and the adoption of the "calm, cool, and collected" expressive facade facilitated her sense of coping with the challenge to her emotional equilibrium upon seeing her friend again. The personal display rule in this case was that if Ruth felt hurt, vulnerable, and/or otherwise threatened, then she would substitute the emotional–expressive behavior that was exactly opposite to what she felt in reality so that she would have at least the *illusion* of feeling relatively strong and invulnerable. Ruth's substitution of a calm or stoic exterior, despite feeling otherwise, is commonly endorsed by latency-age children as an appropriate way to avoid being teased by others (von Salisch, 1991).

Direct Deception in Emotional–Expressive Behavior

In addition to cultural and personal display rules, there is also ordinary deceptive emotional–expressive behavior. The key difference here is a relative lack of social consensus or predictability: One deliberately simulates facial expression, tone of voice, and so forth in a *particular and immediate situation* in order to mislead another about one's emotional experience so as to gain some advantage or to avoid some distinct disadvantage. For example, a girl who has set off the school fire alarm is not likely to express her glee at the commotion caused when in the presence of school authorities, so that she will not be confronted as the possible culprit. This sort of emotional dissemblance that is directly deceptive would not be characterized by *rules* for when it would be employed. One is more likely to use directly deceptive emotional–expressive behavior when there are clear stakes involved in a specific situation. To illustrate, many children suppress their outrage at a teacher's unfairness, because if they did show their anger, they might experience even worse consequences from such a teacher; in contrast, they are likely to express vehemently their outrage at a peer's unfairness, and pity the poor parent who inadvertently appears to be unfair to his or her preadolescent.

SOCIALIZATION OF EMOTIONAL DISSEMBLANCE IN CHILDREN

How do our children acquire display rules and feeling rules, and how do they learn to adopt deceptive emotional–expressive behavior when it is to their advantage? First, as developmental psychologists we have to plead for patience as this question has not been entirely answered by empirical research. However, studies do exist that give us a fair idea as to what children at different ages understand as display and feeling rules, and when it would be strategic to dissimulate one's emotional experience to another. A second point is that typical socialization processes presumably operate in this domain of emotional dissemblance as well, and next we shall briefly describe those traditional socialization methods.

Direct Socialization Methods

By direct socialization we mean that people acquire behaviors that have been rewarded, and they avoid behaviors that have been punished. For example, it is all too common for young boys to experience their fathers' disapproval or temporary rejection if they cry because they had their feelings hurt. (Crying due to injury may be acceptable to many fathers if there is at least some blood dripping somewhere.) Indeed, Fuchs and Thelen (1988) found that sons (preadolescent) did not anticipate showing sadness to their parents, and if they did, it would only be to their mothers. A study with parents undertaken by one of us (Saarni, 1989) confirms what the boys expressed in Fuchs and Thelen's study. Parents were interviewed about how they thought parents in general would react to their children in assorted emotion-eliciting situations. What emerged was that they believed that sons would indeed receive disapproval for expressing a genuine feeling that rendered the child vulnerable (e.g., fear, distress). On the other hand, if daughters expressed their vulnerable feelings genuinely, then parents expected to give them accepting responses.

Consistency of *reinforcement* (reward or punishment) affects considerably the direct socialization of emotional–expressive behavior. Ignoring a child's tantrum may be relatively easy to do at home, but if one's child pulls this emotional stunt in the supermarket, it is considerably harder to ignore the unwanted emotional behavior. Instead, as parents we are then apt to reward such behavior by caving in and buying a sweet to pacify our cranky, screaming child and to avoid our public embarrassment (after all, surely only "bad" parents have children who scream in public). Children learn quickly that tantrum behavior can be very effective at getting what they want.

Another very effective direct socialization method in children's learning how to dissemble how they communicate their emotions to others is peer reaction. Probably most readers can recall some absolutely ghastly situation wherein they expressed how they really felt, and everyone around them responded as though they must be an utter idiot. When children are asked why they would not show their real feelings around other kids, especially if those feelings are what we refer to as vulnerable feelings (fear, anxiety, sadness, distress, etc.), they tell us most often that it would be to avoid being embarrassed or being teased (Saarni, 1979a). Yet children also tell us very emphatically that a youngster who almost always kept all her or his real feelings inside might "consume all her anger, jealousy, whatever, and then one day she'd explode, commit suicide, and get emotionally disturbed" (from an interview with a 13-year-old girl) or at least would be disliked, seen as emotionally maladjusted, or as isolated and hard to get to know (Saarni, 1988). Thus, many children perceive the child who carries emotional dissemblance to an extreme as at the very least peculiar and maybe even self-destructive.

Indirect Socialization Methods

Imitation. By indirect socialization we mean that one learns something by observing others and subsequently imitating their behavior. It is indirect learning in that a time interval occurs between the observation of, for example, someone's emotional–expressive dissemblance, and one's own enactment of the behavior. Children learn by modeling themselves after the emotional expressiveness of their peers and of significant adults. In addition, television provides a source of observational learning about how to manage one's emotional–expressive behavior that may have considerable impact, especially on children who are glued to the TV set for many hours (Saarni & Borg, in press). As an illustration, in a recent study one of us interviewed children about their management of emotional expression in different sorts of social contexts (Saarni, 1991). An 8-year-old boy gave the following answer after being asked whether a boy in a story would modify his facial expression if the interactant (an adult female) were only pretending to be scared at a prank he had pulled: "He would have laughed a little, and if she wasn't laughing, he probably would have stopped." When next asked why he thought this would be the case, he said, "That's what they do on TV shows."

Identification. Under indirect socialization we also include identification, which is essentially modeling one's behavior, feelings, and beliefs after another person with varying degrees of awareness of doing so. Children may identify with a parent and not only develop similar emotional styles and gestures but they may also acquire in this fashion similar strategies of emotional–expressive behavioral dissemblance, for example, masking angry feelings, substituting agreeable or pleasing behaviors for anxiety, minimizing distress, and so forth.

Intriguing is the clinical supposition that some individuals acquire addictive behaviors through identification with an addicted parent, and a crucial part of the identification process may be the incorporation of a way to cope with disturbing emotions by adopting the parent's compulsive behavior, such as becoming dependent on alcohol, for emotional "relief" (Copans, 1989). The addictive behavior functions as a way to change how one feels "on the inside"; the assumption is that the addictive behavior, e.g., compulsive over-eating, chemical dependency, etc., provides temporary relief from experiencing negative feelings such as shame, anger, depression, dread, anguish, and so forth.

Communication of Expectancies. In general, when we have an expectancy that involves an emotion, what the expectancy allows us to do is to anticipate what we will feel in a situation. We may have experienced confusing or ambiguous feelings when we first encountered situation "X," but acquiring an expectancy about how we will feel when "X" recurs means that we have a scheme for labeling or sorting out our previously confusing feelings. The acquisition of emotion expectancies can come from direct experience but, more often than not, emotion expectancies have their origin in social exchange.

Both children and adults respond to what others expect, sometimes defiantly, but more often in the anticipated direction. When a significant adult communicates to a child that he or she will probably feel X, Y, or Z when some event or situation comes to pass, there is a good likelihood that the child will indeed experience the communicated expected feeling. Of course, the expected feeling has to have some plausibility relative to the situation, but once the child does indeed experience something similar to this communicated feeling, then the feeling becomes validated. Upon further repetition the feeling will be internalized by the child as his or her own emotion expectancy when the given situation recurs.

An illustration with adults responding to an emotional expectancy is as follows: One of us recently obtained scuba certification; the communicated and expected feeling was that it would be a wonderful, even euphoric experience. However, this did not conform to the initial reality (i.e., the water was freezing, visibility was only about two meters, there were strong currents, big surf, and generally completely miserable conditions). The positive emotional expectancy was not validated, but the person who had originally communicated the expectation of how one could expect to feel was still considered very credible. So a trip to

Hawaii was planned with participation in scuba diving. Now euphoria and awe were indeed experienced (or was it just nitrogen narcosis?), and a personal emotional expectancy as to what scuba diving could do for one's emotional well-being was firmly ensconced.

Relative to how emotional dissemblance would be influenced by the communication of expectancies, parents may suggest to their children the desirability of dissemblance when they talk about others' emotional *mis*management, as in gossiping about other family members, neighbors, co-workers, etc. in front of their children. Comments such as, "She just couldn't keep her act together and burst into tears," or "He really blew it when he stormed out like that," communicate to children the undesirability of genuine expression of emotion in particular situations or with particular people. As some readers may recognize, children are likely to be extremely attentive to such overheard conversations about the emotional experiences of others, especially if the speaker is relishing his or her story-telling and condemnation of the emotional mismanagement in question (see also Miller & Sperry, 1987).

Peers also communicate expectancies about the "appropriate" way to express one's feelings when they tease another child for his or her genuine expression of emotion. Older children and adolescents may spend considerable time dissecting the behavior of peers and adults to determine whether they are living up to the "acceptable" and expected norms for emotion management (e.g, "Oh, he's such a dork," or "Her parents are original Neanderthals"). These "cutting dissections" communicate quite clearly to the interactant what the expectations are for managing one's emotional–expressive behavior.

COGNITIVE DEVELOPMENT AND EMOTIONAL DISSEMBLANCE

There are several cognitive insights that children must have at their disposal in order to dissemble their emotional–expressive behavior. Chief among these are, first, understanding that how something appears on the surface is not necessarily the same as what lies within and, second, being able to generalize certain abstract qualities about different social relationships and coordinate them with strategies of social–emotional behavior (e.g., expression of genuine emotion is more often accepted and expected in close relationships). We will discuss these two cognitive developmental prerequisites in turn.

Appearance and Reality

By the time they enter school, children generally understand that how one looks on the outside does not necessarily reflect how one feels on the inside. Thus, one's facial expression can be misleading about the actual emotional state being experienced. By age six many children can provide complex justifications for how appearances can conceal reality—in this case, the genuine emotion felt by an individual. Harris and Gross (1988) examined young children's rationales for why story characters would conceal their emotions by adopting misleading facial expressions. A significant number of the six-year-olds interviewed gave very complex justifications that included describing the intent to conceal feelings and to mislead another to believe something other than what was actually being experienced (e.g., "She didn't want her sister to know that she was sad about not going to the party"). Children younger than six can readily adopt pretend facial expressions, but they are not likely to be able to articulate the embedded relationships involved in deliberate emotional dissemblance. These embedded relationships refer to how the self wants another to perceive an apparent self, not the real self. In other words, by age six children readily grasp that emotional dissemblance has as its basic function the creation of a false impression on others.

Recognition of Salient Contextual Cues

Early work by social scientists who studied nonverbal communication had determined that adults varied their nonverbal expressive behavior according to who was the dominant one in an interaction and also according to how close the relationship was (e.g., Mehrabian, 1972). Typically, the nondominant person was more likely to control his or her expressiveness when interacting with a more dominant individual. In close relationships nonverbal expressive behavior was likely to be less controlled and emotions more often genuinely revealed. As a downward extension of this research into childhood, one of us conducted a study of school-age children to examine how they took into account status (Were the interactants equal in status or did they differ?) and affiliation (Was the relationship between the interactants a close one or not?) as they predicted whether story characters' emotional–expressive behavior would be genuine or dissembled (Saarni, 1991). In addition, emotional intensity (strong versus mild feelings) was included as a cue that influenced whether emotional displays were thought to be controllable or not.

The children's responses indicated that they did indeed take into account status similarity or difference, and degree of closeness of relationship, in predicting whether facial expressions would be genuine or dissembled. But if the feelings were very intense, they were often predicted to be genuinely expressed, even though the story character had a lower status and there was little closeness in the relationship with the other story character. In terms of age differences, from age 6 to 12, all children were aware that intensity of emotion and status difference between interactants would influence the protagonist's facial expression; however, older children were more likely to also take into account degree of affiliation between the characters as a factor that influenced whether facial expressions would be genuine or dissembled.

The children were also asked to justify their predictions about facial expressions, and when these were analyzed the most common rationale was to avoid negative interpersonal consequences. However, the variety of rationales increased with age, such that by age 10–12 years, children gave a rich mixture of rationales, ranging from concerns about others' well-being to the desirability of observing norms and conventions, as the reasons why facial expressions were thought to be either genuine or dissembled. Perhaps the point to make here is that children are keenly aware of the interpersonal effects that facial expressions have, and that certain social contexts "require" dissemblance while others are more appropriate for genuine expression of emotion.

MOTIVATION FOR EMOTIONAL DISSEMBLANCE

There appear to be four main categories of reasons why children are motivated to dissemble the expression of their feelings (Saarni, 1979b). Given that most human behavior has multiple determinants, similarly any given instance of emotional dissemblance may have more than one of these motivational categories underlying it. These four motivation categories are also discussed in the order in which they are hypothesized to appear in children's behavioral repertoires (Saarni, 1979b).

The first category is to avoid negative outcomes, as succinctly illustrated by a 6-year-old boy's response to an interview: "He wouldn't show that he thought it [a trick played on another child] was funny, because he'd be scared that the kid would beat him up." This was the sort of rationale mentioned above that was the most frequently offered as a justification for expressive dissemblance.

The second motivation category for dissemblance is to protect one's self-esteem or to cope more effectively with how one feels. An 8-year-old boy said the following: "He could show that he could stand up to stuff like that," in reference to being the target of criticism. When we adopt personal display rules, we may have as our motive the desire to protect our vulnerability, our self-image, or our self-esteem. In this boy's comment what may be alluded to is being able to control stoically one's feelings, despite the threat to self-esteem implied by being criticized.

The third motivation category concerns norms and conventions; these are the cultural display rules that provide us with consensually agreed upon scripts for how to manage our emotions. A couple of 9- to 10-year-old children's responses illustrate their notions of what are norms for emotional dissemblance: "You can't yell at a grown-up" and "You should apologize, even though you don't feel like it." Parenthetically, children may readily articulate culturally accepted scripts for emotional dissemblance, but that does not mean that they will actually perform such scripts, such as apologizing when they would rather not.

The fourth motivation category for expressive dissemblance is to regulate relationship dynamics. This motive appeared most often in preadolescent children's justifications for expressive dissemblance in the research described above. Several of their responses follow: "He didn't want to let the other kids down, so he didn't show his disappointment [at losing the game that he had coached]"; "A friend would know that she felt sorry deep down inside but couldn't show it just then"; "She didn't want to make him feel bad, so she didn't show she was disappointed [upon receiving an undesirable gift from her grandfather]." Concern for others' well-being is a prominent theme among such rationales and is generally associated with relatively close relationships or the desire to increase the closeness of a relationship.

These four categories of why we may be motivated to dissemble the expression of our feelings are not necessarily exhaustive, but they all have one significant feature in common: They are concerned with interpersonal consequences, and it is the varying nature of these social consequences that yields the differences among motives. Even the self-esteem motive for dissemblance does not occur in a social vacuum, for the self is embedded in a history of social relationships.

SOCIAL COMPETENCE AND WELL-BEING: THE NEED FOR EMOTION MANAGEMENT

By the elementary school years, children experience many social encounters in which they feel it is necessary to manage their feelings and their expressive behavior. For example, many of the games that children enjoy between 5 and 10 years of age revolve around the dissimulation of emotions. Not getting angry at the child who obstructed their way in board games like Parchesi or Sorry and pretending to have a great hand in card games challenge children to regulate what they feel and how they express their emotions to others. Even learning to be a "good sport" can be thought of as acquiring the strategies necessary for hiding the frustration and anger felt over losing a game. Masking some of the pride felt after winning a contest has likewise to be learned: Crowing over one's victory is often considered to be immature and thoughtless. The notion of fair play reminds children and adults alike that in disputes the fairness of the procedure has to take precedence over an individual's feelings. In order to comply with this rule, individuals have to manage their emotions in assorted ways.

School-age children often seek out occasions to practice and elaborate their emotion management skills. In such social transactions children have to strike a balance between what they genuinely feel and what is expected by their play partners or by the game at hand. Children also learn that one does not lie to friends (Selman, 1980), and that keeping a secret from a friend is viewed as a sign of distrust. Preadolescent friends insist, "You have to tell me because I'm your friend!" But when friends feel anger or envy toward one another, the rule of honest disclosure comes into conflict with another rule in close relationships, which is to spare the friend's feelings. Appreciation of the friend or fear of rejection calls for inhibiting some of these disturbing negative feelings so as not to hurt another's feelings.

How do girls and boys solve this dilemma between consideration and self-disclosure in a conflict with their friends? This question was addressed in a study that observed the facial expressions of preadolescent children playing a computer game with their best friend, who at this age is almost always of the same gender. The computer game was rigged so that when it broke down it appeared as though one child had not been attentive or skillful enough. In arguing with their friends the girls were inclined to use a double-ended strategy: They blamed their partners verbally, yet gave them a particularly cordial smile, often simultaneously with the verbal reproach. When watching the videotape records of these exchanges, it seemed as if the reproaching girl wanted to reassure her friend that they were still friends. Boys tended to solve the conflict differently: They avoided conflict by expressing few reservations in words, but at the same time they showed more signs of tension, such as touching themselves on their faces or bodies and wiggling in their chairs (von Salisch, 1991).

We do not know if the girls' smiles were intentionally put on, but they did function to maintain the equilibrium of the friendship. These findings suggest that communication occurs on different levels, and the line between intentional dissemblance and habitual social behavior is very hard to distinguish. That the dissemblance is well-practiced is evident from an observation made in this study. One girl seemingly made a mistake in the game, and contempt was visible in her partner's facial expression. However, within a fraction of a second, the partner smiled and said, "Oh, this can happen to anyone." It was clear that the verbal utterance did not reflect her contempt, and her smile was dissembled. What was amazing was the speed in which the dissimulation occurred and the facility that this girl had in expressing both a relationship-nurturing comment and a smile. By preadolescence children seem to have had extensive practice in tailoring their self-presentations such that the intention to deceive is blurred in the day-to-day experience of close relationships.

Sociologist Arlie Hochschild (1983) has pointed out that many relationships are based on the exchange of feelings. An example is the traditional parent–child relationship: Parental love and care is given and children respond with love and filial respect. Whether the feelings are actually felt may not be as important is what is displayed: When children talk back to their parents or hostilely challenge them, the violation of the "rule" for filial respect often provokes considerable anger from the parent. Parents expect that their children will not lie to them, but children may put on false emotional fronts because they fear punishment when under suspicion for some transgression. Many young children believe that their parents can literally read their minds and their hearts, and when children begin to understand that their parents' insight is limited, they may feel relieved (and perhaps a little sad).

Children do indeed on occasion mislead their parents, but this does not usually mean the beginning of a career as a liar or "con man/woman" but rather a test of emerging skills in being able to regulate and manage one's feelings (Ekman, 1989). If children need to establish themselves as separate persons who control what parts of their "inside" they want to disclose to others, then it is not surprising that they select their family for the first stage of rehearsal of internal control and establishment of a private sphere.

In sum, children demonstrate social competence when they can regulate how they express their feelings with others, learning to care for the well-being of those who are close to them by inhibiting some of their negative emotions so as not to hurt the other's feelings. Learning how to manage emotions also contributes to children developing a private domain of the self, a part of themselves to which they control the access or exposure of others', with the result that emotion management broadens their ability to cope with interpersonal conflicts and disappointments.

MALADAPTIVE EMOTIONAL DISSEMBLANCE

From the broadest perspective, emotional dissemblance appears to be adaptive in that virtually all cultures, Western and non-Western alike, have rules or conventions about how, when, and with whom to express one's feelings. It is this plasticity of emotional–expressive behavior that permits emotional dissemblance, which in turn provides the communicative maneuverability needed by individuals to negotiate their way through the maze of social relations that we all encounter. The preceding discussion of motives for emotional dissemblance and the need for emotion management as part of social competence also indicates why this fluidity of emotional–expressive behavior is strategically useful and, hopefully, adaptive. Thus, avoiding negative outcomes and promoting more positive ones will generally be adaptive, as would observing one's culture's norms and conventions for emotional management. Protecting one's self-esteem allows one to cope with emotionally taxing situations, and being able to take into account the well-being of others as a reason for not expressing how one really feels provides for social cohesion. But lest this discussion sound as though all emotional dissemblance is desirable, we turn now to when emotional dissemblance becomes maladaptive.

When emotional dissemblance is used rigidly or indiscriminately, it subverts the adaptive fluidity of emotional–expressive behavior. Simultaneously, the interpersonal consequences of rigidly applied emotional dissemblance become dysfunctional. If one dissembles the expression of one's emotions (or even some emotions) most of the time, then one's relationships with others become impaired. This occurs because those with whom one interacts (e.g., spouse, partner, friend, co-worker, etc.) predicate their transactions with oneself based on what one has falsely communicated about one's internal emotional state. It is our belief that where the greatest toll will be taken is in close relationships; intimacy becomes distorted when excessive false impressions are indiscriminantly applied to our exchanges with those we want to be able to love.

Drawing upon clinical literature, especially marital counseling (e.g., Bradbury & Fincham, 1987), we will describe several specific ways in which emotional dissemblance may become maladaptive. Our examples will focus on adults rather than children, for these maladaptive features of emotional dissemblance are the *outcome* of socialization processes over time. However, given that we are developmental psychologists, the reader ought to bear in mind that parent–child relationships are also influenced by parents' dogmatic or inflexible use of emotional dissemblance toward their children, and this may be a contributing cause to the eventual acquisition of maladaptive emotional dissemblance by the children so affected.

Chronicity

With this term what we want to describe is the maladaptiveness that occurs when emotional dissemblance is chronically used across different situations and different relationships. For example, many adult children of alcoholic parents find that in adulthood they have difficulty establishing intimate relationships because they chronically suppress their expression of feeling vulnerable. As children, having to cope with the frequent emotional upheaval caused by alcoholic parents, the adoption of a chronic "poker face" may have helped them to feel as though they were achieving some semblance of stability and to avoid negative consequences. But what may have been useful and adaptive emotional dissemblance in childhood becomes dysfunctional in adult close relationships. The expression of genuine emotions in many respects defines a relationship as close or intimate in that mutual trust is presumed in order for one to reveal one's emotional vulnerability. Chronically dissembling one's emotions will make it difficult to develop and maintain intimate relations and will cause frequent misunderstandings.

Inflexibility

Related to chronic use of emotional dissemblance is the idea of inflexibility. By this we refer to dissemblance being used without distinguishing among the different emotions that are experienced. Thus, no distinction is made whether one dissembles the expression of one's sadness, one's anger, or one's happiness. A bleaching of emotional expressivity is the result, and that may be what occurs when we encounter a truly boring person. Their flat affective mask conceals all emotional variability, and the unintended social consequence for such an individual is that others avoid them. When our own emotional expressivity is not reciprocated, it becomes easier to withdraw from such people; they are hard to get to know.

There are also conventional roles that may "require" highly stereotyped expressive behavior or masks of blandness. Some sales personnel appear to look this way (but perhaps they really are feeling bored), and occasionally a mask of agreeable smiling appears to be perpetually plastered on "high society" women. While such examples are not necessarily maladaptive instances of indiscriminate emotional dissemblance, they still have the social consequence, perhaps now intended, of keeping others at a distance.

Egocentricity

When egocentricity dominates one's emotional dissemblance, it means that one believes that one's own perspective is shared by everyone else. This can rapidly lead to failures in communication, for if one believes that one's interactant is pretending (when she or he is not), then one responds in light of that mistakenly presumed dissemblance. An example of how this happens in the home is when parents chronically project emotional dissemblance onto their child, in spite of the child's attempts to communicate genuine feelings, because the parents themselves also chronically dissemble their expression of their real feelings. Discounting children's fears, invalidating their sadness over losses, and generally trivializing their intense feelings are common instances of egocentric projections of parents believing that their children are exaggerating their emotional display and thus dissembling their true emotional state.

Excessive Eccentricity

This last form of maladaptive emotion management may be less frequently encountered, because it would have to develop in a person through unusual socialization experiences, not normally encountered in parent–child relationships. It refers to highly idiosyncratic usage of emotion management in social situations, such that no one knows what is being communicated emotionally or can figure out what impression the individual is trying to convey. Perhaps it is analogous to a personal display rule taken to such an extreme that others are not likely to realize what one is experiencing.

A clinical example may be found in adolescents and adults who as children had been severely abused. Twenty-year-old Susan was seen as a client in a college counseling center with her presenting problem as feeling lonely and isolated in the college community. As her life story was revealed, the counselor found out that she had been chronically molested by her stepfather from about age 9 to 14, when she left home to live with an aunt. Her mother was an alcoholic and was both unavailable and unable to protect Susan. Susan had a history of relationships with abusive boyfriends, was on the verge of flunking out of college, and had no social support system. In therapy she presented a facade of "everything's OK" and seemed unconcerned about academic failure, unaffected by a beating she had received from a boyfriend (and was unwilling to press charges), and generally not inclined to pursue goals that reflected a healthy self-interest. Her experience of emotions appeared vague, as though they were tangential to her life. Her style of emotion management was eccentric in that it was extremely difficult for the therapist to perceive what were significant emotional experiences for her. What emotions she did describe did not seem to fit what would be commonly expected within some particular situation (e.g., she appeared indifferent toward the black eye received from her boyfriend). The clinical prognosis for Susan seemed equivocal until the therapist undertook several hypnotic strategies that used metaphors involving feelings of humiliation and hiding when one feels ashamed (see also Lewis, 1991). Susan did indeed view herself as "damaged goods" and felt profoundly humiliated by her history of sexual abuse and victimization. After some months of therapy, she gradually began to redefine herself and became active in a community group for incest victims (which also provided her with a much needed support system).

Such cases as Susan's often reveal childhoods in which victimized children acquire strategies for coping with abuse by dissociating themselves from the trauma and pain inflicted on them. They may not have developed an integrated self, and in adulthood the emotional fragmentation may manifest itself as a more general pseudo-insensitivity to pain and suffering, an emotional depersonalization, whether directed toward the self or toward others. Obviously relationships are negatively impacted, for dissociation functions like eccentric emotional dissemblance: Others flounder about (such as Susan's therapist above), trying to figure out what is going on emotionally within such an individual when they attempt to respond to such dissociative emotional–expressive behavior. For the individual the internal numbness and the external expressive facade make for an emotional experience that feels unreal (Courtois, 1988).

CONCLUSION

In summing up this chapter on the socialization of emotional dissemblance, one may wonder what then are genuine feelings? Are they only those that seem uncontrollable and especially intense? We would argue that the boundary between genuine emotional experience and emotion management is a permeable one, for one has feelings about feelings, and this will lead one to manage one's emotional experience, whether it is an internal emotional state or an external expression of emotion. When we consider that observations of ordinary family life show that children at two to three years of age start to play with the rules governing the expression of emotion (Dunn, 1988), then seen from this perspective, emotional dissemblance loses its moral overtones and becomes one more variant of human interaction. The importance of trust, especially in close relationships, limits the occasions when emotional dissemblance is appropriate, but as we all know, partners in long-term relationships tend to consent to one another's self-presentations and may even strengthen them over time. To put it succinctly: We might be wiser if we knew when others feigned their feelings, but would we be any happier?

References

Blurton-Jones, N. (1967). An ethological study of some aspects of social behaviour of children in nursery school. In D. Morris (Ed.), *Primate ethology*. London: Weidenfeld and Nicolson.

Bradbury, T. N., & Fincham, F. D. (1987). Affect and cognition in close relationships: Towards an integrative model. *Cognition and emotion, 1*, 59–87.

Courtois, C. (1988). *Healing the incest wound: Adult survivors in therapy*. New York: W. W. Norton.

Copans, S. (1989). The invisible family member: Children in families with alcohol abuse. In L. Combrinck-Graham (Ed.), *Children in family contexts: Perspectives on treatment* (pp. 277–298). New York: Guilford Press.

Dunn, J. (1988). *The beginnings of social understanding*. Oxford, UK: Blackwell.

Ekman, P., & Friesen, W. (1975). *Unmasking the face*. Englewood Cliffs, NJ: Prentice-Hall.

Ekman, P. (1989). *Why kids lie*. New York: Scribner.

Fuchs, D., & Thelen, M. (1988). Children's expected interpersonal consequences of communicating their affective states and reported likelihood of expression. *Child Development, 59*, 1314–1322.

Harris, P. L., & Gross, D. (1988). Children's understanding of real and apparent emotion. In J. W. Astington, P. L. Harris, & D. R. Olson

(Eds.), *Developing theories of mind*. (pp. 295–314). New York: Cambridge University Press.

Hochschild, A. (1983). *The managed heart: Commercialization of human feeling*. Berkeley: University of California Press.

Lewis, M. (1991). *Shame: The exposed self*. New York: Free Press.

Malatesta, C., & Havilland, J. (1982). Learning display rules: The socialization of emotion expression in infancy. *Child Development, 53*, 991–1003.

Mehrabian, A. (1972). *Nonverbal communication*. New York: Aldeno Atherton.

Miller, P., & Sperry, L. (1987). The socialization of anger and aggression. *Merrill-Palmer Quarterly, 33*, 1–31.

Saarni, C. (1979a). *When not to show what you think you feel: Children's understanding of relations between emotional experience and expressive behavior*. Paper presented at the meeting of the Society for Research in Child Development, San Francisco, CA.

Saarni, C. (1979b). Children's understanding of display rules for expressive behavior. *Developmental Psychology, 15*, 424–429.

Saarni, C. (1988). Children's understanding of the interpersonal consequences of dissemblance of nonverbal emotional-expressive behavior. *Journal of Nonverbal Behavior. 12*, 275–294.

Saarni, C. (1989). Children's beliefs about emotion. In M. Luszez & T. Nettelbeck (Eds.), *Psychological development: Perspectives across the life-span* (pp. 69–78). North-Holland: Elsevier Science Publishers.

Saarni, C. (1991). *Social context and management of emotional-expressive behavior: Children's expectancies for when to dissemble what they feel*. Paper presented at the meeting of the Society for Research in Child Development, Seattle, WA.

Saarni, C., & Borg, V. (in press). What children learn about emotions from television. In A. Dorr (Ed.), *Television and affect*. Hillsdale, NJ: Erlbaum.

von Salisch, M. (1991). *Kinderfreundschaften*. Göttingen, Germany: Hogrefe.

Selman, R. (1980). *The growth of interpersonal understanding*. New York: Academic Press.

6

Sex Differences in Lying:
How Women and Men Deal with the Dilemma of Deceit

BELLA M. DePAULO
JENNIFER A. EPSTEIN
MELISSA M. WYER

There are ways in which men and women do not differ much in what they want, nor even in what they get, from social life. Both, for example, want and value close friends. And what they want from those friends is not just the sharing of engaging activities but also, more importantly, the sharing of caring and trust (e.g., Sherrod, 1989). Further, during trying times, both men and women are shielded by their friendships from the relentlessness of the stress and the sadness that might ensue if they were facing their troubles alone (e.g., Cohen, Sherrod, & Clark, 1986; Sherrod, 1989).

These similarities are significant. But so are the differences. Though women share activities with their female friends just as men do with their male friends, the activity itself is more the focus of the interaction for the men than it is for the women. Analogously, though both women and men discuss feelings with their friends, the feelings themselves are more the focus of their time together for the women than they are for the men (e.g., Reis, 1986). Relationships, too, are a more prominent theme in women's conversations than in men's (Caldwell & Peplau, 1982). In fact, in most of the topics they choose to discuss, and in the ways they discuss them, women are more revealing of themselves than are men (Aries, 1987; Caldwell & Peplau, 1982; Cozby, 1973; Reis, Senchak, & Solomon, 1985). They are also more supportive of each other (e.g., Aries, 1987; Maccoby, 1990). For example, they are more likely than men to acknowledge each other's points of view and to express agreement with them (e.g., Maltz & Borker, 1983). Also, in their interactions with others, they seem more focused on the other person than men do (Weitz, 1976).

There is depth to this openness and bonding. For the processes that transpire with words also occur without them. That is, women are more open, expressive, and approachable nonverbally as well as verbally (e.g., DePaulo, 1992; Hall, 1984). Their expressions on their faces and the tones of their voices convey their thoughts and feelings more clearly and more dynamically. They smile and gaze at others more than men do, approach others more closely, and touch them more. They are also approached more closely and touched more themselves than are men. Whereas men, more than women, elicit anxiety from the people they meet, women, more than men, elicit warmth (Weitz, 1976).

The differences between men and women in their styles of relating do *not* indicate that men find their social interactions unpleasant or dissatisfying. They do not. But they do judge them to be less gratifying than women judge theirs to be (Reis, 1986). Moreover, the intimacy that women create in their interactions with each other is not something that they alone can appreciate. Both men and women describe their social interactions as more meaningful when they involve a woman than when they do not (Reis & Wheeler, 1992). And for both men and women, the more time they spend interacting with women, the less likely they are to feel lonely. The same cannot be said about time spent with men (Wheeler, Reis, & Nezlek, 1983).

In addition to these qualitative differences, there are quantitative ones. Women spend more of their time with other people than do men (Reis, 1986). And they also spend more of their time thinking about people (McAdams & Constantian, 1983) and reminiscing about important events that occurred in their close relationships (Ross & Holmberg, 1990). In the amount of time they spend with others, then (in their thoughts and in their deeds), and in the way they are when with others, women are indeed the social and emotional specialists in our culture.

What role could deceit play in the lives of these socioemotional experts? Deceit seems, in a way, jarringly at odds with the style we have described and documented. Women, we have claimed, are open and revealing in their interactions with others. Deceit, on the other hand, can be a vehicle not only for hiding oneself and one's feelings, but also for outright fabrication. The "true" self is locked away, and some impostor is unleashed. We have also shown that women are adept at infusing social interactions with intimacy, meaningfulness, and depth. Deceit, in contrast, can be a way of building barriers to intimacy, of keeping others at bay. The esteem, the affection, and the trust that were engendered with caring words, thoughtful probes, and meaningful smiles and glances, can be pierced instantly by a single serious lie, or eroded gradually by a steady trickle of little fibs.

What, then, do women do about deceit? Do they simply eschew lying? Or do they lie in different ways than do men?

WOMEN'S AND MEN'S WAYS OF LYING

Lying More, Lying Less

We wanted to know how often men and women lie, and what kinds of lies they tell, and we did not think it would do simply to ask them this question directly. Instead, we asked 30 men and 47 women to join us as fellow investigators in observing and reporting their own behavior. In this first study (DePaulo, Kirkendol, Epstein, Wyer, & Hairfield, 1991), these men and women were college students. Their primary responsibility was to keep a diary, every day for a week, in which they recorded all of their social interactions, all of the lies that they told during those interactions, and their reasons for telling each lie.

On the average, the participants in this study reported telling about two lies a day. This amounted to a rate of about one lie for every four social interactions. Our first question about these numbers was whether they differed for men and women. They did not. This study suggested, then, that women do not deal with the dilemma of deception simply by refraining from telling lies.

In the diary study, we relied on participants' reports of their own behavior. We think that these reports, though imperfect, are valuable. But we also wanted to see for ourselves the ways in which men and women behave similarly or differently in interpersonal situations which might tempt people to tell lies. We think that there are many, many such situations. The one we chose to look at first was one in which subjects talked to an artist about her work. In this study (Bell, 1991; DePaulo & Bell, 1992), the artists were actually confederates whom we had trained to pose as art students and to behave in a particular way. (Three women alternated in this role.) When we recruited subjects (47 male and 47 female college students), we simply told them that the study was about psychology and art. We then ushered them, one at a time, into a room in which we had displayed close to two dozen paintings. We encouraged them to take their time and look at each one. We then asked them to tell us which two they liked the most, and which they liked the least. Then they wrote down what in particular they liked and disliked about each of the four paintings they had nominated. It was only after they had provided all of this information that we told them that they would be meeting an art student who would ask them about their opinions of the paintings. We told them that the art student would not know which of the paintings they liked most and which they liked least, and that we would not show the art student what they had written about each of the paintings. That way, we (as researchers) would know what they really thought of each painting, but the subjects would not feel compelled to stick to what they had written because the art student would never see that.

We then introduced the subject to the art student, who proceeded to discuss the four paintings with the subject. For each of the paintings, she asked what the subject thought of the painting overall, what the subject specifically liked about it, and what he or she disliked about it. She refrained from offering any of her own opinions. As she opened the discussion of one of the paintings that the subject liked, and one that the subject disliked, she mentioned that the painting was one that she had done herself.

We thought that there were several situations within this study that might seem interpersonally difficult to the subjects, situations that might tempt the subjects to stray from the truth. First, we know from other research that it is often hard for people to say negative things (Blumberg, 1972; Felson, 1980; Tesser & Rosen, 1975). It is hard for them to say what they dislike about each other or even what they dislike about other people, places, and things. Therefore, we thought subjects might tell something other than the complete truth when discussing the paintings they disliked. They might also find it difficult to be totally straightforward when discussing the two paintings that the artist said were her own. The subjects might try to tread more gingerly when discussing those paintings in which the artist had a personal investment. The most difficult moment of all, we thought, would be the one in which the subjects were called upon to discuss the painting that they had described at the start of the study as one that they disliked the most, only to discover later that it was one of the artist's own.

Some of the subjects had no instructions from us as to how to behave in this study. They were simply told to go ahead and discuss the paintings with the artist. We urged some of the other subjects to be very honest in their discussions, noting that it would be more helpful to the artist in her quest to learn more about how art is perceived to hear what they, the subjects, really did think. For the rest of the subjects, we instead urged them to be polite. We said that it was fine to say what they thought of the paintings, but that we did not want the art student to feel bad.

Afterwards, we asked the subjects how sincere they were in their discussions with the art student. We also asked them how much they tried to convince the art student that they really liked each painting, and then compared it to the degree to which they said that they liked each painting at the beginning of the study (i.e., before they knew that they would be meeting an art student who painted some of the paintings). When subjects said that they tried to convey more liking than they felt, they were indicating that they exaggerated their liking to the artist.

In their descriptions of their own behavior, the women did not say that they were always less sincere than the men. But they did say that they were especially insincere when discussing the painting they greatly disliked that was painted by the art student. In that difficult situation of discussing a much-loathed painting with the person who painted it, they were especially likely to have exaggerated their liking for the painting if they had been cautioned not to hurt the artist's feelings.

Would other people see these subjects the same way they saw themselves or are their self-perceptions idiosyncratic? To answer this, we asked two different sets of people to tell us their impressions of the subjects. First, we asked the art students who had interacted with them. Then, we played tapes of the interaction to people who had not been in the original study. Both of these samples thought that the women seemed at least somewhat less sincere than the men, and that they seemed to be exaggerating their liking more than the men. They also noticed special differences between the women and the men in the challenging situation of discussing the detested painting with the artist who painted it. In that condition, the artists thought that the women seemed to be trying to convince them that they liked the painting much more than the men did. They also thought that the women were especially exaggerating their liking for the aspects of that painting that they really did like.

In general, then, both the artists and the other observers agreed with the subjects' own appraisals. All agreed that the women sometimes strayed farther from the truth than did the men, that they often did so by overstating their liking for the paintings, and that they were especially likely to stray from the truth in what may have been the most difficult situation in that study—when talking about the painting they hated that was painted by the artist herself.

Taken together, the two studies suggest that women do not deal with the dilemma of deception by steadfastly telling only the truth. In the diary study, they told just as many lies as the men did, and in the art study, they outdid the men in stretching and reshaping the truth.

There is one example in the literature of a domain in which women may be more truthful than men. In a study in which couples were asked to describe the ways in which they relate events from the past, both the men and the women agreed that men are more likely to alter or embellish details to make a point or to be entertaining, whereas women are more likely to tell their tales accurately (Ross & Holmberg, 1990).

Lying Transparently, Lying Seamlessly

Another way that women can deal with the dilemma of lying, other than by refraining from telling lies (which they seem not to do), is to lie transparently. This might occur if women felt ambivalently about telling lies—we do not know yet whether women feel more conflicted about telling lies than do men. Or it might occur if it were so important to women not to get caught in their lies (because of the interpersonal disruptions that might cause) that they tried too hard and thereby undermined their own attempts.

There is ample evidence that motivation to succeed at lying can undermine the lie (e.g., DePaulo & Kirkendol, 1989; DePaulo, Stone, & Lassiter, 1985a). When people care too much about hiding their lies, they often behave nonverbally in ways that, paradoxically, reveal the lies. In several of the studies in which this motivational impairment effect has been documented, the situations were ones in which the women may have been more invested than the men. For example, they were ones in which the subjects were urged to come across as sincere and likable. And in these studies (DePaulo, Kirkendol, Tang, & O'Brien, 1988; DePaulo, Stone, & Lassiter, 1985b), the women, at least in some conditions, were more likely to be betrayed by their own nonverbal cues than were the men. But we think that there will be situations when men will be especially invested in their deceits, and in those situations, their lies should be more transparent than women's.

In summary, there is as yet not much evidence that women deal with the dilemma of deception by lying ineptly. Across the many studies of sex differences in skill at deceiving, there is no compelling evidence that women lie more transparently than do men (Zuckerman, DePaulo, & Rosenthal, 1981). But in most of those studies, subjects were not highly invested in their lies. When motivation to get away with one's lies increases, lies do become obvious from nonverbal cues. We have seen this happen to women more often than to men, but this could be because the situations we created in our studies caused the women to be more concerned than the men with making a good impression.

If women do not lie less often than men, and they do not lie more openly (transparently) than men, then perhaps there are other ways that women lie differently than men. For example, there could be differences in the styles of lying, in the content of the lies, or in the motivations for lying. Those are questions we are addressing as we continue our work in this area.

LYING AS SERIOUS BUSINESS

For each of the lies that subjects recorded in their diaries, we asked them to tell us how distressed they felt at three points in time: before they told the lie, while telling the lie, and after telling the lie. The men and women were similar to each other in generally reporting only very mild levels of distress about their lie-telling experiences. But while telling their lies, women became somewhat more uncomfortable than did the men. After the lie was told, men reported feeling a bit less distressed than they had felt while telling the lie. But women did not. They continued to feel the same slight twinge of discomfort after the lie as they had felt during it (Wyer, 1989). It was as if they could not quite let go of the lie.

We thought that the emotional aftermath of lie-telling for women was especially intriguing because so many of the lies reported in the diaries were so pedestrian. What would happen when the lies were much more serious?

To understand more about momentous lies, we conducted a study focused solely on serious lies (DePaulo & Kirkendol, 1991; Kirkendol, 1986). Sixty-eight college students—28 men and 40 women—participated. Each of them told us about the most serious lie they ever told to anyone, and the most serious lie that anyone ever told to them. We asked them many questions about these experiences, including questions about the person who lied to them or to whom they told their lie, and questions about how they reacted to the lie.

The pattern of findings that emerged from this study suggested that these serious lies were serious business to both the men and the women, but perhaps more so to the women. The women seemed more engaged by these experiences and more upset by them (see also Levine, McCornack, & Avery, 1991). For example, when talking about the episodes in which they were the ones who told a serious lie to someone else, they described themselves as more anxious, tearful, and apologetic than did the men. When the roles were reversed and they were the ones who were being duped, women described themselves as more actively involved in testing their suspicions than did men. They, more often than men, said that they scrutinized the suspected liar's behavior, looked for other kinds of evidence, and talked to other people about their suspicions. At the key moment when the lie was finally confessed, the women were less likely than were the men to feel indifferent or unconcerned, to pretend that they felt that way, or to pretend that they never suspected anything.

The differences between the sexes did not end at the point at which the lie was revealed. As the diary study led us to surmise, there were important emotional postscripts to these events. The ways that women talked about the experience of being deceived suggested that they may have been more embittered by it than were the men. For example, they more often castigated the persons who deceived them as having told the lie for self-centered reasons. And the more serious the lie was, the more likely they were to impute these egoistic motivations. Unsurprisingly, then, they also reported that one of the short-term effects of the lie was that they and the liar behaved more guardedly toward each other. This tendency for women, more than men, to feel that the lie episode had created this more guarded way of relating to each other was not simply a short-term effect, for they described it as continuing even over the long term. One final piece of evidence also suggested to us that women took these serious lies even more seriously than did men. When we asked the subjects to tell us how often they still think about the lie episode that they described, women, compared to men, said that the matter was more often on their minds.

LYING IN CLOSE AND CASUAL RELATIONSHIPS

Because close interpersonal relationships may in some ways be even more important to women than to men, we thought that the threat lying can pose to those relationships might prove especially worrisome to women. As a result, they might take the lies that they tell to their close friends more seriously than the lies they tell to their casual friends, and this difference might occur even for the mundane kinds of lies that were so often reported in the diary study. If women were especially concerned about the threats to their close relationships that lying could pose, then did they deal with this in the seemingly straightforward manner of simply telling fewer lies to their close friends than to their casual friends? They did do this, but so did the men, and the women did not do it any more than the men did. What did seem to differ between the sexes was their investment in their lies.

For all of the lies that were reported in the diary study, we asked the subjects who had told each one to tell us how serious they thought the lie was, how much planning they had put into it, and how important it was to them to avoid getting caught in the lie. Then we looked at what they had to say about the persons to whom they had told their lies—most importantly, did they describe them as close friends or as casual ones? We thought that all of the subjects would report more investment in their lies told to close friends than their lies told to casual friends, but that women would do this even more than men would. Women did, in fact, show the predicted pattern (Wyer, 1989). For example, when they described the lies they told to close friends, they said that they had planned those lies more carefully than the lies they told to casual friends. The men, though, did not show this pattern at all. Instead, they tended to show a reversal of our predictions, describing the lies told to casual friends in a somewhat more serious way than the lies told to close friends.

SEEING TRUTHS, SEEING LIES

We have seen that there is a warm and accommodating gloss to the way that women lie, when compared to how men lie. (For other discussions of women's accommodating style, see LaFrance, 1981, and Weitz, 1976.) We know that much of this positivity and supportiveness is false because the women have told us so themselves. In the art study, for example, they sometimes admitted to more insincerity than did the men, and they also claimed, in certain conditions, that they had tried to convince the art student that they felt more positively about her paintings than they did in fact.

The data from the art study tell us how women and men behave toward others. We wondered whether women might be similarly positive and accommodating in the ways that they perceive others. For example, do they, more than men, see others in the ways that others prefer to be seen?

Overlooking Lies, Questioning Truths

We went back to the art study once again to help us learn more about the ways that men and women differ in how they perceive others. We showed videotapes of the subjects discussing the paintings with the artists to other men and women, whom we will call "judges." The judges watched the subjects on the tape as they talked about the paintings they liked and the paintings they disliked. However, the judges were not told which paintings the subjects liked and which ones they disliked. We wanted to see if they would sense insincerity as they listened to the subjects discuss different kinds of paintings, including some of the artists' own. And, of course, we wanted to see if the women's sense of insincerity was different from the men's.

Indeed it was. The female judges thought that the subjects were generally more sincere during their discussions with the artists than the male judges thought they were. There were certain kinds of discussions that the women viewed as especially more sincere than the men did. These included discussions about the paintings the subjects really did like, discussions of the paintings the subjects really did like that were painted by the artists, and the discussions involving the subjects who were told explicitly to be polite and avoid hurting the artists' feelings. These were, of course, just those discussions during which subjects were most likely to be saying positive things about the paintings (whether they meant them or not). The female judges accepted these expressions of positivity as basically sincere more than the male judges did.

We also asked the judges directly how much they thought the subjects really did like the paintings and the extent to which they thought the subjects were trying to convince the artists that they liked the paintings (whether they did or not). We found that the men and women did not differ at all in their perceptions of the latter sort of liking, that is, the amount of liking that the subjects seemed to be trying to convey to the artists. But they did differ in their perceptions of the amount of liking they thought the subjects really did feel. The women thought that the subjects felt more liking than the men thought they did. The women, compared to the men, thought that more of the liking that subjects expressed was genuine, and less of it was exaggerated. If it is safe to assume (and we think that it is) that the subjects wanted their expressions of liking to be seen as genuine, then the female judges, more than the male judges, were viewing the subjects as the subjects preferred to be viewed. They were being more accommodating.

This accommodating pattern of females in their perceptions of others is one that we have seen many times in many other studies (Rosenthal & DePaulo, 1979a, b). For example, in one study, we showed male and female judges videotapes of people who were describing people they liked and people they disliked. Sometimes they described those people honestly—when they liked them, they said that they did, and when they disliked them, they said that. Other times, though, they described the people dishonestly. They pretended to like the people they actually detested, and they pretended to dislike the people they actually liked. We asked the judges how much liking they thought the subjects really did feel for the persons they were describing. When the subjects were pretending to like the people they actually despised, the women thought they felt more genuine liking than the men thought they did. This is just like what we found in the art study. Women view other people's overt expressions of fondness as more genuinely positive than men do. The female judges in the person description study were not only more positive in their perceptions of the subjects, but also more accommodating. They saw things the way the subjects wanted them to. When the subjects were pretending to dislike people they actually liked, the sentiment that they want others to believe is the disliking. They are trying to convince others that their feelings are negative, even though they are not. The female judges, more than the male judges, go along with that. They say that the subjects seemed to feel more dislike than the men thought they did. This suggests that it may be more important to women to be accommodating in their perceptions than to be positive. For when others seem to want to be viewed negatively, then that's how women view them.

When women listen to a person who is only pretending to like another person and they say that they think that person's sentiments really are positive, they are overlooking deception. Either they never see the deceit in the first place, or they do see it but close their eyes to it. If women are in fact blind to deceit, it is not because they cannot see. When women are observing people who are not lying, they are much more perceptive than are men about how the people are feeling. In the same person description study, when the speakers were relating their honest descriptions of people they liked and people they disliked, the female judges were much better than the male judges at realizing how much the speakers really liked their favorite people, and how much they disliked their least favorite people. Women, then, are more skilled than men at understanding how others are really feeling when those others are telling the truth; but they are not any better, and sometimes even worse, when others are lying. The theme, again, seems to be accommodatingness to others' wishes. When people are telling the truth, they want their true feelings to be recognized, but when they are lying, they want only their faked feelings to be noticed. And that is just what women do when they observe.

Seeing Faces, Hearing Voices

When people have feelings or attitudes that they would like to hide from others, they try deliberately to be careful about the way they act so those feelings will not "leak" out. They are, of course, careful about what they say. But they are also careful about how they say it. For example, if a man suggests going out for Chinese food to a woman who just went out for Chinese four nights ago and then ate the leftovers for the next three, the woman might still try to act delighted by the suggestion. And if so, she would try to regulate her facial expression so that it seemed to convey the pleasure that she was pretending to feel rather than the disappointment that she really did feel. Most people, including both men and women, do think to monitor their facial expressions so that their faces will show only what they want them to show. They remember to do this because the face is so often the focus of interest and attention in social interaction (e.g., Ekman & Friesen, 1969). When the feelings that people are trying to hide are not terribly intense, they can usually succeed at putting on a facial expression of a different kind of feeling that they want to pretend to be experiencing. That is, when the stakes are not too high, people are usually fairly successful at lying with their faces. If others try to look at their faces to see whether to believe them, they may well be fooled. Instead of seeing what the person really is feeling, they will see what the person is pretending to feel.

The situation is different for other kinds of cues like body movements and tone of voice cues (Ekman & Friesen, 1969). People do not seem to think to be careful about their postures and about the ways that they move their hands and legs and feet to the same degree that they are self-conscious about their faces. They probably do try to control the tone of their voices, but that can be hard to do, and often they do not succeed.

There are important differences, then, in what kinds of behaviors are most likely to convey what people want them to convey, and what kinds of behaviors instead might leak what people are trying to hide. Facial expressions are behaviors that, under ordinary circumstances, can be controlled fairly successfully to convey what people want them to convey. Body movements, and even more so, tone of voice cues, can instead leak the hidden messages. If women wanted to be accommodating in the ways in which they observed other people, then what they might do is to pay attention primarily to behaviors such as facial expressions, because those are the behaviors that are most likely to tell only what others want them to. They would pay less heed to body movements or tone of voice cues. And they certainly would not pick up the fleeting "micromomentary" facial expressions that might last just a fraction of a second but in that flash could contradict the broader, fuller, intended expression and thereby reveal something that was meant to be hidden. Discrepancies, too, would be off limits: If a woman noticed that another person seemed to be conveying contradictory emotions at the same time, as if he were pretending to feel something that he really did not feel, she might just overlook that.

We did a series of studies in which we tested men's and women's preferences for attending to different kinds of behaviors (DePaulo, Rosenthal, Eisenstat, Rogers, & Finkelstein, 1978; DePaulo & Rosenthal, 1979a). We showed them a film of a person who was conveying contradictory feelings. For example, she might seem to have a happy face but her voice might sound sad. Or the reverse might occur—she might seem to have a sad face but a happy voice. We found that both women and men tended to favor the visual information—when indicating how they thought the woman really did feel, they tended to report the feeling that she was expressing in her face or in her body movements more than what she was expressing in her voice. Either they did not much notice the tone of voice information, or they simply trusted it less than, say, the facial cues. This is an accommodating way for observers to act. They are favoring just those cues (i.e., facial cues) that are easiest for people to regulate so that they convey what they want, without leaking what they do not want. It should follow, then, that women show this accommodating pattern of perceiving others even more than do men. And this is, in fact, exactly what we found.

The studies just described show that women, more than men, pay special attention to the behaviors that are most under other people's control. But when they look at such readily-regulated behaviors as facial expressions, are they skilled at understanding the attitudes or feelings that are communicated by those expressions? Are they especially better at this than are men? And how successful are they at reading the kinds of behaviors that they are "not supposed to" read, such as tone of voice cues and micromomentary cues and discrepant cues? To explore this, we showed male and female judges films of facial expressions, of body postures and movements (without showing the accompanying faces), and of facial expressions or body movements that conflicted with tone of voice cues in the emotions they conveyed. We also showed them films of facial expressions that lasted just fractions of a second (comparable to fleeting micromomentary expressions) and we played sound tracks for them in which they could only hear the tone of voice without being able to hear any of the words (which had been muffled or distorted). We found that women were generally better than men at understanding these various nonverbal messages. More importantly, they were especially better than men at understanding the messages that others would want them to understand, the ones that are easiest for people to control. Their biggest advantage over men was in their reading of ordinary facial expressions. They were also better than men at reading body movements and postures, but not as much better as they were at reading faces. At reading tone, they lost more of their advantage still, and still more in trying to read the very brief facial expressions. In trying to determine when messages were or were not discrepant, they sometimes showed no advantage over men at all (Rosenthal & DePaulo, 1979b).

The pattern of women's superiority over men in their ability to understand nonverbal cues is clear. Women are most superior at reading the cues that are easiest for others to regulate so that they convey what they want them to convey. But as cues become more covert and harder to control, women systematically lose their advantage over men, and end up, for certain kinds of cues, having no advantage at all. We found this pattern in the U. S. samples that we tested in our own lab, and we also found the pattern generally to hold across the many other studies in the literature of sex differences in understanding nonverbal cues. But the phenomenon is not unique to the United States. Men's and women's skill at reading facial expressions, body movements, and tone of voice cues has been assessed in 51 samples recruited from 11 different countries (Hall, 1979). The results were impressively consistent with what we had already learned from just our own culture: The women were most superior to the men at reading facial expressions, less superior at reading body movements, and least superior at reading tone.

In some countries, though, the pattern was more striking than it was in others. The differences were not haphazard. Those countries in which women, compared to men, were especially likely to show the accommodating pattern in the way they read nonverbal cues were those in which women seemed to be most oppressed. For example, they were the countries in which there were proportionately fewer women in higher education and fewer women's groups.

Even within the U.S. samples that we studied, not all of the women showed the accommodating pattern, and of those who did, not all showed it to the same degree. Again, the differences were telling. Those who showed the pattern most clearly were those who were uncomfortable with hostility, uncomfortable asking others for help, less socially adroit (i.e., less likely to be shrewd, sophisticated, and success-ful at persuading others by indirect means), and lower in self-monitor-ing (i.e., more likely to just be themselves across situations rather than trying to alter their behavior from situation to situation). Women who are most accommodating in the way they view others, then, seem to be those who do not want to offend or intrude, and who open themselves to others in an almost naive way. They tend *not* to be boastful, manipulative, hostile, or assertive (Rosenthal & DePaulo, 1979a).

We wondered what the interpersonal lives might be like for women who show this accommodating pattern most clearly. One possibility is that these women who seem so meek in their interactions with others will be unpopular and unhappy. But the ways in which these women seem "meek" are actually consistent with conventional standards of sex-appropriate behavior. According to the traditionalists, women *should* be careful not to offend or intrude. If there are rewards for sex-role conformity, then perhaps the women who are more accommodating will be more socially successful.

To determine the interpersonal effectiveness of the high school students we had tested, we asked their teachers to rate each of the students' popularity with the same sex and the opposite sex. With the college students, we asked them to tell us themselves how satisfied they were with their relationships with other people. According to the teachers' perceptions of the high school students, and the college students' perceptions of themselves, those women who were most accommodating in the ways that they read others' nonverbal cues were those who were most successful in their social lives (Rosenthal & DePaulo, 1979b).

LYING ACROSS THE LIFE-SPAN

Childhood and Adolescence

We have focused in our work on sex differences in lying during the late adolescent years. Because of the intensity of interest in mating and dating that occurs during that period of development, we thought that it might be a particularly telling time for the expression of many sex differences—not just those related to lying. The famous anthropologist Ray Birdwhistell (1970) speculated that sex differences in expressive behaviors may become more and more marked over the course of development throughout childhood and early adulthood, but then may decline somewhat after that time.

Our hunches were in accord with Birdwhistell's. The relevant data are somewhat sparse, but those strands of evidence that do exist seem supportive. Beginning with the childhood data, there is evidence for sex differences consistent with those we have reported even in young children. And there is also evidence that these sex differences become more pronounced as males and females approach the late adolescent years.

A few of these studies have been conducted with children as young as three years old. For example, in one study (Lewis, Stanger, & Sullivan, 1989), an experimenter placed a toy behind a three-year-old and left the room, telling the child not to look at the toy until the experimenter returned. The vast majority of these children could not resist; they looked at the toy. Upon returning, the experimenter asked if the child had peeked. More of the boys than the girls truthfully admitted that they had. The girls were more likely to stonewall the question, giving no response at all, not even a nod or a shake of the head. In the diary study that we conducted with adolescents, there were no sex differences in the frequency of reported lies. But in the art study, the women did describe themselves as somewhat less sincere than did the men in certain conditions.

The "no-peeking" situation is so different from the situation we created in the art study that it is difficult to know whether the two can be compared. But there is another kind of paradigm that has been used in studies of children that seems much more comparable to the art study. It involves a situation, first used by Saarni (1984), in which children receive presents that they love (such as candy and money) as a reward for helping an adult with her work. Shortly thereafter, they are asked to help again. But this time, the present they are given is a boring one, more suitable for children much younger than these seven-through eleven-year-olds. How did the children react? It was the girls in the study who more often smiled and beamed at the gift-bearing adult, despite their disappointment. A similar study was conducted with three-year-olds (Cole, 1986), and even at this tender age, the girls pretended to be pleased much more readily than did the boys. It does not seem terribly rash to imagine these three-year-old girls some 14 years later gazing at a painting that they detest, but then telling the artist who painted it how lovely the colors are.

Can we also see in children the beginnings of the pattern of greater female accommodation in ways of perceiving other people's truths and lies? On this matter, we can draw comparisons much more straightforwardly, because the issue has been addressed, and with exactly the same study materials that were used in the studies of late adolescents. In one of these investigations (DePaulo, Jordan, Irvine, & Laser, 1982), sixth, eighth, tenth, and twelfth graders, as well as college students, were shown the videotapes of people describing people they liked or disliked either honestly or deceptively. When the people on the tape were describing their liking and their disliking honestly, the females were much better than were the males at recognizing how much they liked their favorite persons and disliked their least favorite persons, just as they were in the original study (DePaulo & Rosenthal,

1979b) in which the people watching the tape were college students. Also as in the original study, the females were no better than the males at separating the dishonest descriptions from the honest ones; in fact, when asked how they thought the speakers really did feel when they were lying, the females were especially likely to say that the speakers felt the way they were pretending to feel, and not as they really did feel. This pattern in which the females, more than the males, seem to hear what they probably think the speakers want them to hear, was evident at every age level, from sixth grade on up.

We also repeated the study of people's interpretations of facial expressions, body movements, tone of voice cues, and discrepant communications with younger subjects. We did this study cross-sectionally, testing junior high school and high school students as well as college students, and also longitudinally, testing 11- through 14-year-olds one year and then a year later (Blanck, Rosenthal, Snodgrass, DePaulo, & Rosenthal, 1981). In both parts of the study, we found evidence for the development of sex differences in accommodation. As they grew older, the females became relatively better than the males at understanding the more overt cues (such as facial expressions) and relatively worse than the males at noticing the kinds of cues that people might not like them to notice, such as discrepancies in communications.

Middle and Late Adulthood

To suggest that sex differences in lying might be especially glaring during the late adolescent years is to propose not only that such differences might become stronger as children grow older, but also that they might become weaker as men and women progress into adulthood. We know of no published data that are relevant to this important question. We are beginning to work on this issue in our lab, using the same diary methodology that we used in our study of undergraduates. We hope that we and others will have much more to say about these issues in the near future.

SUMMARY AND CONCLUSIONS

We have emphasized the ways in which women in particular deal with the dilemma of deception. We have focused more on women than on men because what we know about men's and women's interpersonal lives led us to suspect that lie-telling might be more problematic for women. In their everyday lives, women appear to be more people-oriented than men. They spend more time with other people, they think about them more, and they talk about them more. Their style of interacting with others is to be more open, more expressive, more supportive, and more approachable than men. They add intimacy and meaningfulness to the lives of both the women and the men with whom they interact.

In that lies can be interpersonally distancing and destructive, it might seem that the only way women can manage to be so supportive and so intimate is by resolutely telling nothing but the truth. But this is not what they do. By their own admission, they tell just as many lies as do men, and sometimes they even shade the truth more than men do. The differences between men and women, then, are in the ways that they lie. Women's lies seem to contribute to their supportiveness. They lie warmly and protectively.

A less compassionate way to put this is that women seem to achieve some of their supportive qualities by way of deceit. At least some of the times when women are being protective of other people's feelings, they are simply lying. Men are less supportive in those ways, but also more truthful.

It is not only women's ways of lying to others that is accommodating, but also their ways of perceiving the truths and lies told by others. Women's legendary sensitivity to the thoughts and feelings of other people has important limits. Women are most sensitive to the thoughts and feelings that others are *not* trying to hide. When other people want to keep their feelings to themselves, women often seem politely to overlook any signs of those feelings that might be apparent to them. They appear to see and hear mostly only what others want them to.

Yet the story of women and deception is not only one of sweetness and light. When they are the targets of deceit, especially when they are the targets of very serious deceits, women are neither particularly kind nor particularly docile. They actively scrutinize the suspected liar and the situation until the lie is definitively discovered or confessed. Then they point a recriminating finger at the liar, and refuse to mute their emotions. They have a more guarded relationship with the liar afterwards, and continue to mull over the episode long after it has ended.

Lying is often regarded as a manipulative and morally reprehensible act that is used callously to further the liar's self-interests. And indeed, lies sometimes are used selfishly and even exploitatively. However, we believe that lies that are self-serving in baldly instrumental ways are less common, both for women and for men, and less interesting psychologically, than the subtle lies that are often told to protect the privacy, the feelings, and the self-esteem of oneself and others. Lies told for these purposes—particularly when told to protect other people—are more apt to be regarded as indicative of social skill and interpersonal sensitivity than of moral depravity. And it is women, more than men, who seem to specialize in telling these socially sensitive lies.

Acknowledgments

The research in this chapter was supported by a research grant and a Research Scientist Development Award from NIMH to the first author. We thank Kathy Bell and Toni Wegner for their helpful comments on an earlier version of this chapter.

References

Aries, E. (1987). Gender and communication. In P. Shaver & C. Hendrick (Eds.), *Review of personality and social psychology: Vol. 7. Sex gender* (pp. 149–176). Newberry Park, CA: Sage.

Bell, K. L. (1991). *When is it hard to tell the truth? Strategies for conveying difficult information.* Unpublished Master's thesis, University of Virginia.

Birdwhistell, R. L. (1970). *Kinesics and context.* Philadelphia, PA: University of Pennsylvania Press.

Blanck, P. D., Rosenthal, R., Snodgrass, S. E., DePaulo, B. M., & Zuckerman, M. (1981). Sex differences in eavesdropping on nonverbal cues: Developmental changes. *Journal of Personality and Social Psychology, 41,* 391–396.

Blumberg, H. H. (1972). Communication of interpersonal evaluations. *Journal of Personality and Social Psychology, 23,* 157–162.

Caldwell, M., & Peplau, L. A. (1982). Sex differences in same-sex friendship. *Sex Roles, 8,* 721–731.

Cohen, S., Sherrod, D., & Clark, M. (1986). Social skills and the stress-protective role of social support. *Journal of Personality and Social Psychology, 50,* 963–973.

Cole, P. M. (1986). Children's spontaneous control of facial expression. *Child Development, 57,* 1309–1321.

Cozby, P. (1973). Self-disclosure: A literature review. *Psychological Bulletin, 70,* 73–91.

DePaulo, B. M. (1992). Nonverbal behavior and self-presentation. *Psychological Bulletin, 111,* 203–243.

DePaulo, B. M., & Bell, K. L. (1991). *Lying kindly.* Unpublished manuscript.

DePaulo, B. M., Epstein, J. A., & Kirkendol, S. E. (1991). Everyday lying in the post-adolescent years. Unpublished data.

DePaulo, B. M., Jordan, A., Irvine, A., & Laser, P. S. (1982). Age changes in the detection of deception. *Child Development, 53,* 701–709.

DePaulo, B. M., & Kirkendol, S. E. (1989). The motivational impairment effect in the communication of deception. In J. Yuille (Ed.), *Credibility assessment* (pp. 51–70). Belgium: Kluwer Academic Publishers.

DePaulo, B. M., & Kirkendol, S. E. (1991). *Serious lies.* Unpublished manuscript.

DePaulo, B. M., Kirkendol, S. E., Epstein, J. A., Wyer, M. M., & Hairfield, J. G. (1991). *Everyday lies in adolescent life.* Unpublished manuscript.

DePaulo, B. M., Kirkendol, S. E., Tang, J., & O'Brien, T. (1988). The motivational impairment effect in the communication of deception: Replications and extensions. *Journal of Nonverbal Behavior, 12,* 177–202.

DePaulo, B. M., & Rosenthal, R. (1979a). Telling lies. *Journal of Personality and Social Psychology, 37,* 1713–1722.

DePaulo, B. M., & Rosenthal, R. (1979b). Ambivalence, discrepancy, and deception in nonverbal communication. In R. Rosenthal (Ed.), *Skill in nonverbal communication* (pp. 204–248). Cambridge, MA: Oelgeschlager, Gunn, & Hain.

DePaulo, B. M., Rosenthal, R., Eisenstat, R. A., Rogers, P. L., & Finkelstein, S. (1978). Decoding discrepant nonverbal cues. *Journal of Personality and Social Psychology, 36,* 313–323.

DePaulo, B. M., Stone, J. I., & Lassiter, G. D. (1985a). Deceiving and detecting deceit. In B. R. Schlenker (Ed.), *The self and social life* (pp. 323–370). New York: McGraw-Hill.

DePaulo, B. M., Stone, J. I., & Lassiter, G. D. (1985b). Telling ingratiating lies: Effects of target sex and target attractiveness on verbal and nonverbal deceptive success. *Journal of Personality and Social Psychology, 48,* 1191–1203.

Ekman, P., & Friesen, W. V. (1969). The repertoire of nonverbal behavior: Categories, origins, usage, and coding. *Semiotica, 1,* 49–98.

Felson, R. B. (1980). Communication barriers and the reflected appraisal process. *Social Psychology Quarterly, 43,* 223–233.

Hall, J. A. (1979). A cross-national study of gender differences in nonverbal sensitivity. Unpublished manuscript, Northeastern University.

Hall, J. A. (1984). *Nonverbal sex differences: Communication accuracy and expressive style.* Baltimore: The Johns Hopkins University Press.

Kirkendol, S. E. (1986). *Serious lies: First person accounts.* Unpublished Master's thesis, University of Virginia.

LaFrance, M. (1981). Gender gestures: Sex, sex-role, and nonverbal communication. In C. Mayo & N. M. Henley (Eds.), *Gender and nonverbal behavior.* New York: Springer-Verlag.

Levine, T. R., McCornack, S. A., & Avery, P. B. (1991). Gender differences in emotional reactions to discovered deception. Paper presented at the annual meetings of the International Communication Association, Chicago, IL.

Lewis, M., Stanger, C., & Sullivan, M. W. (1989). Deception in three-year-olds. *Developmental Psychology, 25*, 439–443.

Maccoby, E. E. (1990). Gender and relationships: A developmental account. *American Psychologist, 45*, 513–520.

Maltz, D. N., & Borker, R. A. (1983). A cultural approach to male-female miscommunication. In J. A. Gumperz (Ed.), *Language and social identity* (pp. 195–216). New York: Cambridge University Press.

McAdams, D. P., & Constantian, C. A. (1983). Intimacy and affiliation motives in daily living: An experience sampling analysis. *Journal of Personality and Social Psychology, 45*, 851–861.

Reis, H. T. (1986). Gender effects in social participation: Intimacy, loneliness, and the conduct of social interaction. In R. Gilmour & S. Duck (Eds.), *The emerging field of personal relationships* (pp. 91–105). Hillsdale, NJ: Erlbaum.

Reis, H. T., Senchak, M., & Solomon, B. (1985). Sex differences in the intimacy of social interaction: Further examination of potential explanations. *Journal of Personality and Social Psychology, 48*, 1204–1217.

Reis, H. T., & Wheeler, L. (1991). Studying social interaction with the Rochester Interaction Record. In M. Zanna (Ed.), *Advances in experimental social psychology* (pp. 269–318). New York: Academic Press.

Rosenthal, R., & DePaulo, B. M. (1979a). Sex differences in accommodation in nonverbal communication. In R. Rosenthal (Ed.), *Skill in nonverbal communication* (pp. 68–103). Cambridge, MA: Oelgeschlager, Gunn, & Hain.

Rosenthal, R., & DePaulo, B. M. (1979b). Sex differences in eavesdropping on nonverbal cues. *Journal of Personality and Social Psychology, 37*, 273–285.

Ross, M., & Holmberg, D. (1990). Recounting the past: Gender differences in the recall of events in the history of a close relationship. In J. M. Olson & M. P. Zanna (Eds.), *Self-inference processes: The Ontario Symposium, Volume 6* (pp. 135–152). Hillsdale, NJ: Erlbaum.

Saarni, C. (1984). An observational study of children's attempts to monitor their expressive behavior. *Child Development, 55*, 1504–1513.

Sherrod, D. (1989). The influence of gender on same-sex friendships. In C. Hendrick (Ed.), *Review of personality and social psychology. Vol. 10: Close relationships.* Newberry Park, CA: Sage.

Tesser, A., & Rosen, S. (1975). The reluctance to transmit bad news. In L. Berkowitz (Ed.), *Advances in experimental social psychology* (Vol. 8, pp. 194–232). Orlando, FL: Academic Press.

Weitz, S. (1976). Sex differences in nonverbal communication. *Sex Roles, 2*, 175–184.

Wheeler, L., Reis, H., & Nezlek, J. (1983). Loneliness, social interaction, and sex roles. *Journal of Personality and Social Psychology, 45,* 943–953.

Wyer, M. M. (1989). *Everyday lying in close and causal relationships.* Unpublished doctoral dissertation, University of Virginia.

Zuckerman, M., DePaulo, B. M., & Rosenthal, R. (1981). Verbal and nonverbal communication of deception. In L. Berkowitz (Ed.), *Advances in experimental social psychology* (Vol. 14, pp. 1–59). New York: Academic Press.

7

Looking at Oneself in a Rose-Colored Mirror:
The Role of Excuses in the Negotiation of a Personal Reality

SANDRA T. SIGMON
C.R. SNYDER

And he said, Who told thee that thou wast naked?
Hast thou eaten of the tree, whereof I commanded thee
   that thou shouldest not eat?
And the man said, The woman whom thou gavest to be
   with me, she gave me of the tree, and I did eat.
And the LORD God said unto the woman, What is this
   that thou hast done? And the woman said, The serpent
   beguiled me, and I did eat.
          —Gen. 3:11–13. King James Version

SALE!!!! NEW, IMPROVED METAPHOR
ROSE-COLORED MIRRORS

(Get a rebate for turning in rose-colored glasses)

The preceding two events, though separated in time by thousands of years, have influenced our thoughts regarding the use of excuses and how we alter negative feedback about ourselves. We call this process of giving an excuse and thus aiding in the continuation of our positive self-image, reality negotiation. First, let us explain why these two events introduce this chapter.

One of the most famous excuses appears in the biblical story of Adam and Eve. Just as Adam and Eve had difficulty in accepting responsibility for their actions, we often find ourselves in situations where we choose to separate ourselves from what we have done. Conclusion: Giving excuses often allows us to look better in others' eyes, as well as continuing to look good in our own mind's eye.

The second event, the sale, perplexed us. Having been so content with our glasses, we were reticent about change. Was it a new fad, the "in" purchase of the 1990s? Of course, we were pleased at the recycling effort and the sale price. We decided to investigate a little further and try out the mirror. As we looked into our respective mirrors, we were struck by the fact that we saw only ourselves in a positive light, not others. We did not have to hassle with taking the glasses on and off; the mirror was easy and convenient. Conclusion: The rose-colored glasses metaphor was no longer sufficient to describe the process that we engage in as we positively bias incoming information about ourselves. For those of you who missed the sale, we have written this chapter to convince you of the appropriateness of our new metaphor in this psychic bargaining process that characterizes most individuals.

Some interesting unexpected findings came out of the depression literature a few years ago. Normal individuals (i.e., those who were not depressed) were found to *overestimate* the amount of control, responsibility for positive outcomes, and their strengths relative to their weaknesses in many experiments (Beach, Abramson, & Levine, 1981). In short, most of us look at the world through "rose-colored glasses" *when we view ourselves*. It should be emphasized, however, that our lenses for viewing other people are *not* so tinted; that is, most people do not overestimate the virtues of other people. Perhaps a more succinct metaphor is called for in order to describe this process. Our choice would be the "rose-colored mirror." With a mirror, of course, we are looking at ourselves and not others, and the rose color assures that a positive image will be reflected back to us. Using the "rose-colored mirror" metaphor, in the present chapter we will present the argument that having a positive biased perception of reality characterizes most healthy individuals.

We will first discuss the process of reality distortion and the adaptiveness of this process. Looking at the "rose-colored mirror" further, we present excuse-giving (in its various forms) as a prime example of the reality negotiation process. Next, we address the confusing relationship between lies and excuses. Furthermore, the process of self-deception is examined as a means of reducing discrepant personal information and as an aid in the negotiation of reality. In summary, we present some pros and cons of excuse-giving as it relates to the reality that we negotiate for our personal selves.

SELF THEORY AND REALITY NEGOTIATION

In the last decade, there has been a revival of interest in the self, most notably in the area of self-concept (Arkin & Baumgardner, 1986; Epstein 1973, 1980; Markus & Wurf, 1987). The self-concept is increasingly viewed as not only a reflection of our present behavior, but as a mediator and regulator as well. In this respect, the self-concept can be conceptualized as the structure that represents the self as well as the dynamic process influencing interpersonal and intrapersonal behavior. Extending this analysis to a more abstract level, a theory about the self reflects basic assumptions, core beliefs, and corollaries representing less central beliefs (Snyder, Irving, Sigmon, & Holleran, 1992). For example, throughout this chapter we will refer to two main assumptions that we believe most individuals hold about themselves: (1) "I am a good person," and (2) "I am 'in control' most of the time." These core assumptions underlying typical self theories are formed over time and represent a collage of perceptions and images about the self across a multitude of situations.

Imagine your self theory as a house with many levels and rooms. We like our home to be relatively unchanging in most respects, yet we often engage in enhancing and protective projects. Locking doors and windows, paying insurance premiums, painting and maintenance of the structure are all examples of enhancing and protective behaviors we engage in with respect to our home. Similarly, our self theory needs protection and enhancement. Just as we only want visitors (and often ourselves) to see certain rooms of our house, we only want our "clean," "good and in control" self to be seen. Our self theory is vulnerable to attack from without as we are constantly bombarded with conflicting personal information about the self. Ways to protect and maintain our self theory are presented next.

The problem arises when we are faced with some disconcerting or incongruent feedback about our self theory. What happens when a core belief is challenged by new information? To maintain a sense of balance about our self beliefs, the new information must be revised or transformed in some manner. Rather than calling a demolition crew to tear down our psychological home, we engage in a reality negotiation process. Accommodating this new conflicting information about the self into a form that is more consistent with our core beliefs represents a negotiated reality (Snyder et al., 1992).

Perhaps it may be useful at this point to provide an example of how the reality negotiation process works. The behavior: a student is caught cheating on an exam. The excuse: the student explains that he/she has never done anything like this, will never do so again, and was just too stressed by the material. The negotiation of reality: the student thinks of him/herself as a "good" person, with the anomalous event of having done a "bad" thing by cheating on the exam. The student has to account for the cheating to others and to him/herself. How can the student acknowledge the "bad" deed and still maintain that he/she is basically a good person? The student reasons that this was a one-time action and that he/she was too stressed by the material. By giving extenuating circumstances, the student is able to maintain the belief that he/she is basically a "good" person. Even a "good" person can occasionally do a "bad" thing. This process not only helps to modify conflicting information about the self, but also helps reduce negative feelings that arise in the situation. Thus, the transformed information represents a somewhat slanted truce between what we perceive about ourselves and what we believe others will not seriously dispute or contest. In response to threatening information about the self, the reality negotiation process serves to maintain and protect our self theory.

What is the driving force behind the reality negotiation process? We have mentioned the powerful function that this process can serve in maintaining and protecting self theory. The core beliefs of being a "good and in control" person are similar to two basic human motives: maintaining a positive self-image, and maintaining a sense of control (Snyder et al., 1992). A lot of human interpersonal and intrapersonal behavior is fueled by these two motives. To preserve our core beliefs when confronted with conflicting information, we must bias that information in such a way that does not challenge our self theory. In addition, reality negotiation allows us to decelerate the rate of change, especially in regard to corollary assumptions (i.e., more minor beliefs) about ourselves. Through reality negotiation processes, we have more time to incorporate new information and sustain a cohesive, functional theory of self (Snyder, Higgins, & Stucky, 1983).

CONSTRUCTION OF THE MIRROR IMAGE: APPRAISAL PROCESSES IN REALITY NEGOTIATION

We propose that the negotiation of personal reality is carried out on two primary dimensions: linkage-to-act and valence-of-act. These two dimensions reflect appraisal processes stemming from a cognitive schema composed of the organized knowledge surrounding the self. Linkage-to-act "reflects the degree to which the person believes that he/she is yoked to a particular act or outcome" (Snyder, 1989, p. 134). In other words, linkage refers to how much we believe we are connected to an event in a causal way. Valence of act "reflects the degree to which any outcome is considered to be negative or positive" (Snyder et al., 1992, p. 277). In other words, valence refers to how we judge events on a good to bad continuum.

When we are confronted with events that relate to or challenge our self theory, the appraisals of linkage and valence are very much intertwined. For example, when confronted with a positive personal event, we tend to see ourselves as strongly linked to such an outcome. For a very negative personal event, on the other hand, we attempt to lessen the linkage. There are many possible combinations of linkage and valence elements involved in our appraisal processes of events as we construct our mirror. For example, if your college basketball team won a game, you might say, "*We* won last night." If your team lost, you might say, "*They* lost" (see Snyder, Lassegard, & Ford, 1986). We tend to increase our connection to positive events and decrease our linkage to negative events. On a more personal level, you might not have reported all of the income to the IRS that you received from tips in your job as a waiter. After having done this "bad" thing, you decrease your linkage to the event and negative aspects of it by saying that "everyone does it."

As we develop into adulthood, we come to understand the causal role that we play in our environment. We learn how much responsibility to assume for our actions and when to assume said responsibility. Thus, our perceptions of what causes events (i.e., causal reality) are influenced by our experience of the causative and associative links between events that continue to influence our developing theory of self. For example, Johnny (who is 2 years old) may be told, "Don't hit your brother." As Johnny gets older, his mother may say, "Don't hit your brother, you may hurt him." Johnny learns that there is a causal link between his hitting and hurting his brother. This experience becomes even more pronounced if there is some physical evidence of the hurt. Johnny's acceptance of responsibility for his actions is influenced by statements such as, "I know you must have hit your brother, he's crying," or, "I know you didn't mean to hit him." Thus, our parents and significant others begin to shape our concept of personal causality, when to assume varying levels of responsibility.

The valence-of-act appraisal reflects our perception of where we place an outcome on a positive to negative continuum. More often than not, valences of "good" and "bad" are the ones that most affect our self theory, and particular "bad" outcomes evoke the reality negotiation process. To take full responsibility for a bad outcome can be potentially damaging to our core self beliefs. Later, we will discuss how excuses can function to soften the impact of such situations and bias our perception of reality as it relates to our self.

Through our developing years, we are continuously taught to discriminate between good and bad. By the processes of reward and punishment, we typically learn to increase our responsibility or linkage to more positive acts and to decrease our linkage to more negative acts (Snyder et al., 1992). As mentioned previously, the motives for linkage and valence appraisals come from our need to preserve self-esteem and to maintain control. Most of us have biased appraisals of ourselves in that we attribute higher self-esteem and more control to ourselves than would be warranted by the situation (Beach et al., 1981; Taylor & Brown, 1988). Thus, the biased appraisal process involved in reality negotiation helps reinforce the self theory of being a "good and in control" person. This scenario probably fits most individuals confronting normal stressors in their lives. It appears to be adaptive in that individuals who view themselves as "good and in control" people are seen as being more well-adjusted and healthy on many psychological measures (Snyder & Higgins, 1988a; Taylor & Brown, 1988). Thus, looking at a rose-colored mirror seems to be beneficial for preserving and maintaining our self theory.

LOOKING INTO THE MIRROR: EXCUSES AND REALITY NEGOTIATION

Most of us probably do not want to admit that we give excuses and that we are very proficient at doing so. Excuses have a negative connotation in our society and at first glance, it may seem maladaptive to use them. However, the truth is closer to the fact that we utilize them constantly, and ultimately they may preserve and/or enhance our self theory. The giving of an excuse may allow us to gaze longer into the mirror and reinforce that cherished image of the "good and in control" person.

How Did I Become so Adroit at Giving Excuses?

There may be no quick and easy answer to the question of why we do the things we do. After years of practice, however, we can verbalize "reasons" for most of our actions. Early in our development, we learn from parents and others that if we give a "good" enough answer to the Why question, we can often escape punishment. At the very least, we learn that the external audience demands an explanation of us. Parents will often supply the answer to the Why question for us. "Why did you hit your sister . . . I know you didn't mean to hurt her," or "She must have said something to make you angry." As we grow older, the external as well as our own internal audience helps refine and discriminate appropriate explanations for our behavior. As our self theory develops, we find that it becomes ever more important to be viewed by others and by ourselves as being consistently "good and in control people." As children, we are reinforced for associating ourselves with more positive outcomes (e.g., "That's a good girl/boy"). Individuals who develop a negative self theory (associated with more negative outcomes), on the other hand, may be characterized later by more dysfunctional or abnormal behavior (e.g., clinically depressed individuals).

Increasingly, our verbal behavior about our actions or inactions needs to be in alignment with our self theory. Our excuse-giving repertoire expands and becomes honed to the tune of self-protection and self-enhancement. This process begins early in childhood and continues throughout our life-span. We all have a basic need to preserve and protect the view we have of ourselves. Yet, this self view is constantly being challenged by new and often discrepant information about ourselves. Whenever we are asked the Why question, we immediately become defensive, our self-protection mode is activated, and reality negotiation in the form of excuse-giving begins.

The What, When, and Why of Excuses

The What. Excuses are defined as actions or explanations that lessen the negative impact of an act and help to maintain a positive perception of oneself (Snyder et al., 1983). When we find ourselves in the situation of giving an excuse, it is often because of some negative attribution about ourself concerning some act, action, or outcome with which we are connected. We go through an appraisal process, evaluating our degree of linkage and where the outcome falls on a positive to negative valence continuum. We automatically assess our connection to it and where it falls on the good-to-bad dimension. For example, imagine that your petition for mandatory recycling was turned down. You would evaluate your contribution to the proposal; Was it something I did or failed to do that resulted in the defeat? Or was the defeat more related to the make-up of the city council who typically vote against environmental concerns? Often, the appraisal process allows us to "save face" by engineering reasonable excuses such as, "It's that city council, they're behind the times where recycling is concerned."

The When. As the appraisal of the situation nears the more negative side of the valence continuum and our sense of linkage increases, we are more likely to engage in the reality negotiation process of excuse-giving. When we experience any potentially threatening feedback about one of our actions, we are more likely to offer an excuse. Bad acts often mean bad people, and this represents a direct threat to our self theory. For example, you make a comment about how you can't stand people who have cosmetic plastic surgery. You learn later that your dinner companion has had plastic surgery on his nose. You don't want to hurt anyone's feelings (because you are basically a good person) so you apologize (i.e., make a particular type of excuse) for your comment, "I didn't realize you had an operation, I must have come across like a real buffoon." We should point out that excuses typically come "after-the-fact"; however, they can be anticipatory. For example, you may feel that you will not do well on an assignment. You preface your acceptance of the assignment by saying, "I'll do the best I can even though I have not been feeling well." Your self-image is protected no matter how the assignment turns out. If you do well on the project, others will think even more positively of you, due to the fact that you did well despite your illness. If you do not do well, then your illness becomes the excuse, or reason for your bad performance.

The Why. Excuses can function to diminish the perceived link between the self and the bad act and/or diminish the badness of the act. Not only can excuses preserve our "rosy" view of ourselves, but they also can preserve the rosy view that we want others to have of us. In many cases, we can immediately decrease the negative impact of our action while saving face with others. If only for the benefit of hearing ourselves verbalize an excuse, we can begin to repair any tears in our self theory and reconstruct our own version as to why we did or did not do something. Regardless of how effective our excuses are to the external audience, we are immediately reinforcing our view of what transpired. Excuses are a part of our social network, and unless they are of an extreme nature (e.g., "My dog ate your invitation and I couldn't remember the address"), they serve as a glue to hold that network together. We would much rather hear the excuse of "I'm sick" than to hear "I really can't stand you or your parties." This latter point brings up an important distinction between lies and excuses that we will examine next. At times, the difference between a lie and an excuse may be slight. Several dimensions are presented that may aid in the discrimination of the two forms.

MIRROR IMAGES? LIES AND EXCUSES

In order to discern any differences between lies and excuses, it is useful to examine these two concepts on dimensions involving definitions, acceptability, responsibility, and function.

Definitions

According to Webster, a lie is "an assertion of something known or believed by the speaker to be untrue with intent to deceive." The verb to lie is "to make an untrue statement with intent to deceive." Our definition of excuses is "actions or explanations that lessen the negative implications of an actor's performance, thereby maintaining a positive image for ourself or others" (Snyder et al., 1983, p. 45). According to Webster, to excuse is "to make apology for or to try to remove blame from." Notice that with the noun and verb form of lie, there is the commonality of intent to deceive. This is not necessarily true in all cases of excuses. Certainly, some types of excuses, such as denial or alibis, can be conceptualized as lies. Most excuses, however, are probably based in "reality," at least as seen by the excuse-giver. Later, we will discuss the relationship between self-deception in excuse-giving, as well as other-deception.

Acceptability

Excuses seem to come to our lips much more easily than lies. As children, we learned that lies are punished more frequently and are less socially acceptable. As we grow older, lies are socially censored when the audience recognizes the intent to deceive. On the other hand, we are taught the process of excuse-giving as an alternative to lying, even though it is not openly acknowledged by our parents and others. Excuses seem to hold the social fabric together as well as our own internal fabric. Does the external audience's awareness of the circumstances affect whether a statement is viewed as an excuse or a lie? Whether the external audience has access to the facts, and how familiar they are with the content will help determine if the statement is labelled as a lie or as an excuse. Certainly lies have the more negative connotation of the two (although excuses are viewed negatively), and if we have a choice in the matter of labelling, we will choose the label of excuse. With regard to acceptability, therefore, the excuse is more socially sanctioned than a lie.

Responsibility

In most types of excuses (with the exception of denial and alibis), there is an attempt to accept some level of linkage and therefore responsibility for the action. This is true even when the excuse-giver tries to minimize the linkage to the act. In excuse-giving, the speaker may offer extenuating or mitigating circumstances that will decrease responsibility, but there is an acknowledgment of the causal link. In the case of lies, there does not appear to be any attempt to accept responsibility when one is linked to a bad outcome. Rather, there is the implicit assumption of intent to deceive. The very nature of most excuses suggests a recognition of responsibility and an intentional effort to elicit forgiveness for the bad behavior. For example, after the Tower Report was released in 1987 regarding the Iran–Contra scandal, President Reagan made the following statement: "A few months ago I told the American people I did not trade arms for hostages. My heart and best intentions still tell me that it is true, but the facts and evidence tell me that it is not" (Reagan, 1987, p. A18). Later on, the President stated "As I told the Tower board, I didn't know about any diversion of funds to the Contras. But as President, I cannot escape responsibility" (Reagan, 1987, p. A18). In this example, it is clear that the President is trying to distance himself from an outright lie, and at the same time come across as accepting responsibility for some portion of the action. Again, the President is trying to explain that he had no intention of harming anyone and offers excuses (e.g., his heart and best intentions) for the discrepancies in facts.

Function

We have discussed the importance of excuses in protecting and enhancing self theory as well as preserving our standing with others. Lies, such as denial or alibis, might function in the same way. However, not all lies are in response to some action committed by the speaker. A lie may be offered when no "reasons" are warranted for a bad outcome. "I am 25 years old." "I would love to come to your party." Although these lies may enhance self theory or increase social standing, they do not attempt to minimize linkage or decrease the negative valence of some action. Lies seem to cover a much broader area of verbal behavior, although at times they may function similarly to excuses. The essence of the excuse appears to be in the call to the excuse-giver to give reasons for an action. In summary, lies may function to keep the hearer ignorant of the facts while excuses are offered to "enlighten" the hearer (i.e., both oneself and others). Next, we present some common excuse forms that relate to linkage and valence dimensions.

FORMS OF EXCUSES

Linkage-Related Excuses

"*I didn't do it.*" Excuses of this form attempt to negate the fact that the person had anything to do with the particular bad act or outcome (Snyder et al., 1983). The least sophisticated type in this category is *denial*, often recognized by others as lies. "I was at a movie at the time of the crime," and "I did not eat all of the ice cream" are examples. These types of excuses imply a complete break with any acceptance of linkage to the action and, through external verification, can very well be completely discredited.

A somewhat more sophisticated version of denial is the *alibi*. This type of excuse is often pertinent in legal situations and again, no linkage is admitted in regard to the bad action. "I was out all day with my niece." "At that time, I was at the museum." As in the case of denial, there is some potential for verifying the link between the excuse-giver and the act.

Blaming refers to the type of excuse that points the finger of linkage and responsibility toward someone or something else. "My dog ate the bill." "My husband forgot to tell me that you called." This type of excuse can backfire, however, especially if the person blamed (e.g., a co-worker or spouse) is in a continuing relationship with the excuse-giver or is a "superior" (Higgins & Snyder, 1989).

These three types of "I didn't do it" excuses may be less successful than "Yes, but" responses (described subsequently) in interpersonal situations, but nevertheless they may provide some aid to support the excuse-giver in reducing his/her association with negative outcomes and in protecting his/her self theory.

"*Yes, but.*" Although the "yes" part acknowledges some linkage to the action, the "but" part helps decrease the linkage between the excuse-giver and the action (Snyder et al., 1983). The critical part of the excuse hinges on the "but" that forms the basis for extenuating circumstances to follow. The mitigating conditions elaborated in this form of excuse will aid in decreasing the linkage to the excuse-giver.

A familiar type of the "Yes, but" excuse is "*I couldn't help it*" (Snyder et al., 1983). In this instance, the excuse-giver attributes the reason for the action to some force outside his/her own will. Attributions are often made to fate, luck, physical or mental illness, alcohol or drugs, or demons. "I was possessed," "It must be God's will," and "It was the luck of the draw," all point to decreasing linkage by attributing causality to an external force. In essence, the excuse-giver is saying that he/she would not ordinarily do this type of thing *but* some force overpowered his/her will.

The "*I didn't mean to*" type of excuse attempts to decrease linkage between the action and the excuse-giver by focusing on intention. Excuses of this type often contain or are followed by an apology. "I didn't mean to hurt your feelings, I was just playing around." "I didn't mean to spill wine on your carpet, I'm sorry." In these instances, the appeal involves acknowledging the link to the action but attempts to decrease that linkage with an appeal to lack of intention. Therefore, a positive self-image can be preserved because there was no "intent" to hurt, harm, or deceive, and the excuse-giver can remain a "good" person.

The last form of the "yes, but" excuse refers to the "*It wasn't really me*" type. Again, the excuse-giver attempts to decrease the linkage between an act and his/her self. In this case, the excuse contains reference to a different part or aspect of the self that is linked to the bad act. "It was the alcohol talking." "My temper got away from me." The part(s) of the self referred to in the excuse are responsible and known for "bad" acts, but do not represent the "real" person.

"Yes, but" forms of excuses are usually more successful than "I didn't do it" forms in interpersonal situations because the excuse-giver does acknowledge some linkage to the bad action. In addition, there is social reinforcement for "owning up" to the situation. "Owning up" may enhance the self theory as well. Excuses of this form are more socially acceptable and probably represent a large number of excuses offered by the general populace as they negotiate reality.

Valence-Related Excuses

Excuses of the "It wasn't so bad" form attempt to minimize the negative valence of the act. The excuse-giver acknowledges linkage, but attempts to reframe the "badness" of the act by reinterpreting the outcome in a more positive light.

Minimization excuses attempt to change the valence of the bad act in a direct way by focusing attention on more minor aspects of the action (Snyder et al., 1983). "It was only a small dent." "I only got one D." The operative word in this type of excuse is "only." This implies that this situation is not typical for the excuse-giver and does not represent the usual outcome. In addition, critical information may be left out of the excuse to further minimize the negative outcome, such as "I didn't spend all the money," when in fact the person left only pennies in the account.

As mentioned earlier, we can often avoid punishment if we give a "good enough" explanation or reason for our actions. *Justifications* are called reasons by the excuse-giver and seem plausible to the external audience. "She did it first." "I was paid to do it." With justification, the excuse-giver decreases the negative valence of the act, enhancing standing with others and protecting the self theory.

In *derogation*, the excuse-giver attempts to decrease the negative valence of an act by employing excuses that downgrade the content or context. Examples include "He doesn't know anything," "When he stared at me, he was asking for it," and "They don't have feelings anyway." The implication in the excuse is that the action cannot be so "bad," because the recipient was somehow not deserving of anything better. In this instance, the excuse-giver attempts to divert attention away from the "badness" of the act by derogating the external source in order to protect self theory.

The "It wasn't so bad" forms of excuses function to minimize the negative connotations associated with the excuse-giver's action. Justification and minimization are probably more successful in interpersonal situations because there is some responsibility acknowledged. Although derogation may assist the excuse-giver in negotiating reality to protect self theory, there may be costs if the excuse-giver is in ongoing relationships with those persons who are derogated.

WHO'S LOOKING AT THE MIRROR: SELF-DECEPTION AND EXCUSES

A common view of excuses is that they are ways of deceiving others. Although the external audience plays a large role in the development, maintenance and often fine art of excuse-making, excuses also can function as a way of deceiving ourselves (Snyder, 1985; Snyder & Higgins, 1988a). We would define self-deception as a reality negotiation process in which a person holds two conflicting self beliefs, with the more negative one being less in awareness (Snyder, 1985). In order to help resolve the conflict of holding two antithetical beliefs about the self (e.g., the "good/in control" self is linked to something bad), reframing and transforming strategy excuses are offered.

Reframing

Through a self-deceptive resolution, excuse-givers attempt to lessen the negative impact of actions for which they are responsible. Inherent in reframing strategies is the excuse-giver's lack of perception of the act being that "bad" (Snyder, 1985). Minimization, justification, and derogation would be excuse types that serve to decrease the negative valence of an action. In other words, "I'm still a good person because the act was not that bad." The two disparate self beliefs thus are resolved by an excuse that reframes the negative valence into a more neutral one.

Transforming

To resolve the conflict between the two self beliefs, "I am a good person and I am responsible for a bad act," the excuse-giver transforms the second belief to "I am less or not totally responsible for a bad act" (Snyder, 1985). Of course, the "I didn't do it" type of excuse does not really transform responsibility, because the self belief is "I did not commit a bad act." The "yes, but" type of excuse more cleanly fits the self-deceptive process of transforming responsibility for a bad act. The excuse-giver admits linkage to the action and generates mitigating circumstances as to why he/she should be held less responsible.

To aid in the transforming of linkage and accompanying responsibility, an excuse-giver will often appeal to consensus and consistency types of information in the development of his/her excuse (Snyder et al., 1983). A consensus-raising excuse may be offered that indicates others would have acted in a similar way, given the situation. "Everybody does it." "Most people would have done the same." Excuses like these are designed to appeal to the masses in that others would have behaved in a like manner. The consistency-lowering excuse strategy appeals to the unique or less frequent situation. If we act in a manner that is inconsistent from our usual self, then we are viewed by others as being less responsible for the bad act. "I didn't mean to" or "I didn't try" point to situation-specific acts that are not representative of our normally stable and positive behaviors. If an excuse-giver can transform the linkage to the bad act from total to some reduced level, then she/he has successfully engaged in self-deception and/or other-deception ("I am a good person who is less responsible for a bad act"). When the valence of the bad act has been reframed and/or responsibility transformed, the excuse-giver has paved the way to resolving antagonistic self beliefs and deceiving the self.

We should mention that there is a residual dilemma in offering excuses. Not only has the "good/in control" person committed the original bad act to which he/she has been linked, but this person has done a second socially unacceptable thing (or one that has a bad reputation), that is, has engaged in excuse-making. Even though society promotes the giving of excuses, it also attaches negative connotations to these "weak and silly" ploys. Thus, there is a second bad act to which the excuse-giver can be linked. Individuals who have been "caught" giving excuses will often not realize that they were giving them and offer this defense, "It's not an excuse, it's the truth." Thus, the final step in the self-deceptive process of excuse-giving involves the perception that we have not given excuses, but that we have given explanations or reasons for the bad act.

Is the Rose-Colored Mirror Working?

Often we give excuses to deceive others, but not in an intentional way. Maybe we do not want to hurt someone's feelings or we feel we must give a more socially acceptable reason for our action or inaction. Deceptive socialization in the form of excuse-giving is pervasive and begins early in our life. For example, Johnny may not like a classmate and may not want to attend the classmate's birthday party. Johnny overhears his mother telling the classmate's mother that Johnny cannot attend the party because they are going to the zoo that day. As our self theory develops, we also feel a need to give ourselves reasons for our actions in order to reduce conflicts with our core beliefs. But is this self-deceptive process always within our awareness, and do we "intentionally" engage in it?

We are not always able to judge with accuracy how "bad" our action was or to what degree we are ultimately responsible (Snyder et al., 1992). Because most of our interpretations of events are biased and our memories are inaccurate, it may be reasonable to assume that the self-deceptive process of excuse-giving is not always intentional and in total awareness. In essence, we are not forced to "excuse" deceiving ourselves.

In addition, giving excuses allows us to recognize our limitations and to take risks (Snyder et al., 1983). As small children, most of us held the belief that we were a major causal force in our world. This all encompassing responsibility changes through the years with the developing skill of excuse-giving. We learn that we can take risks, attempting tasks or acts that may be beyond our skills at present. Taking chances in new areas is possible because we can fall back on excuses if we are unsuccessful (e.g., "This was just my first time, you can't expect me to do it perfectly").

When the Rose-Colored Mirror Breaks

We have talked mostly about the successful nature of excuses in deceiving the self and others. However, there are some instances in which excuse-giving can become detrimental. Extremism in any form can undermine and diminish the positive aspect of excuses. A person who offers too many or too few may be socially ostracized, which may have a negative impact on one's self theory. In some instances, a person may literally become their excuse, culminating in a self-fulfilling prophecy (Snyder & Higgins, 1988b). For example, a person labelled as an alcoholic may become so entrenched in the "disease" excuse that his/her adaptive coping becomes severely limited. A depressed person may not be expected to perform as well as others. If these lowered expectations continue, the depressed individual may not be given opportunities to succeed or be responsible. Thus, the label of depression may lead to the "living" of the excuse and its continuation, possibly hospitalization. At this point, excuses may not be as effective in resolving the discrepant information that impacts core beliefs. Although there are occasions when the self-deceptive nature of excuses becomes debilitating, it should be emphasized that, in moderation, excuses are an adaptive accommodation of reality that generally work well in intrapersonal and interpersonal situations.

REFLECTIONS ON THE ROSE-COLORED MIRROR

By distorting and even altering conflicting new information, we are able to preserve the "rosy" view that we have of ourselves. The process of excuse-giving further enhances our self-view and enables us to deceive others and ourselves. Even though we do not like to think of ourselves as excuse-givers, we successfully use them to our advantage. We are shaped and trained to use excuses, yet we do not want to acknowledge their use. We engage in excuse-making so effortlessly and with such proficiency that we do not often perceive that we are doing so. We continue to protect and enhance our self theory with this self-deceptive process in an artful negotiation of reality.

Our argument throughout this chapter is that people do *not* see everything in this world in a positive light, but most people do seem to view *themselves* positively. This reasoning has led us to conclude that the proverbial rose-colored glasses may be more accurately supplanted by the rose-colored mirror metaphor. Indeed, when it comes to the negotiation of personal realities, most people carefully attend to their rose-colored mirrors. In this process, excuses help us make certain that our reflections remain bright and shiny.

References

Arkin, R. M., & Baumgardner, A. H. (1986). Self-presentations and self-evaluations: Processes of self-control and social control. In R. F. Baumeister (Ed.), *Public self and private self* (pp. 75–97). New York: Springer-Verlag.

Beach, S. R. H., Abramson, L. Y., & Levine, F. M. (1981). Attributional reformulation of learned helplessness and depression. In J. F. Clarkin & H. I. Glazer (Eds.), *Depression: Behavioral and directive intervention strategies* (pp. 131–195). New York: Garland STPM Press.

Epstein, S. (1973). The self-concept: Or, a theory of a theory. *American Psychologist, 28,* 404–416.

Epstein, S. (1980). The self-concept: A review and the proposal of an integrated theory of personality. In E. Staub (Ed.), *Personality: Basic issues and current research* (pp. 82–132). Englewood Cliffs, NJ: Prentice-Hall.

Higgins, R. L., & Snyder, C. R. (1989). Excuse gone awry: An analysis of self-defeating excuses. In R. C. Curtis (Ed.) *Self-defeating behaviors: Experimental research, clinical impressions, and practical implications* (pp. 99–130). New York: Plenum.

Markus, H., & Wurf, E. (1987). The dynamic self-concept: A social psychological perspective. *Annual Review of Psychology, 38,* 299–337.

Reagan, R. (1987, March 5). Transcript of President Reagan's speech, March 4, 1987. *New York Times,* p. A18.

Snyder, C. R. (1985). Collaborative companions: The relationship of self-deception and excuse making. In M. W. Martin (Ed.), *Self-deception and understanding* (pp. 35–51). Lawrence, KS: Regents Press of Kansas.

Snyder, C. R. (1989). Reality negotiation: From excuses to hope and beyond. *Journal of Social and Clinical Psychology, 8,* 130–157.

Snyder, C. R., & Higgins, R. L. (1988a). Excuses: Their effective role in the negotiation of reality. *Psychological Bulletin, 104,* 23–35.

Snyder, C. R., & Higgins, R. L. (1988b). From making to being the excuse: An analysis of deception and verbal/nonverbal issues. *Journal of Nonverbal Behavior, 12,* 237–252.

Snyder, C. R., Higgins, R. L., & Stucky, R. J. (1983). *Excuses: Masquerades in search of grace.* New York: Wiley-Interscience.

Snyder, C. R., Irving, L. M., Sigmon, S. T., & Holleran, S. (1992). Reality negotiation and valence/linkage self theories: Psychic showdown at the "I'm OK" corral and beyond. In L. Montrada, S. H. Filipp, & M. Lerner (Eds.), *Life crises and experiences of loss in adulthood.* Hillsdale, NJ: Erlbaum.

Snyder, C. R., Lassegard, M. A., & Ford, C. E. (1986). Distancing after group success and failure: Basking in reflected glory and cutting off reflected failure. *Journal of Personality and Social Psychology, 51,* 382–388.

Taylor, S. E., & Brown, J. D. (1988). Illusion and well-being: A social psychological perspective on mental health. *Psychological Bulletin, 103,* 193–210.

8

Lying to Yourself:
The Enigma of Self-Deception

ROY F. BAUMEISTER

Lying and deception may have infiltrated many features of how people relate to others. But what about lying to oneself? Is this pervasive? Does it work the same way as lying to others? What are its peculiar advantages and disadvantages?

This chapter will take a close look at self-deception. It begins with the basic question of how it is even possible to lie to oneself. Next, it examines the relationship between lying to others and lying to oneself. Although the mechanisms are different, lying to others is often a vital part of lying to oneself. (In other words, the self is more readily fooled if others are fooled too.) Lastly, it will try to weigh the costs and benefits of lying to oneself.

HOW IS SELF-DECEPTION POSSIBLE?

In ordinary lying, the liar misleads the dupe about some information that the liar knows and the dupe does not. Self-deception, however, requires that the same person be both the liar and the dupe. That, in turn, means that the same person must both know something and simultaneously not know it. For this reason, a number of thinkers have advanced the argument that self-deception may be logically impossible (see Sartre's, 1953, critique of Freud; also, more recently, Sackeim & Gur, 1979).

On the other hand, self-deception seems so widespread and familiar that it is hard to dispute that it happens. Everyone can cite instances of wishful thinking, of overconfidence, of people who refuse to recognize their own faults (often despite a penetrating awareness of the same faults in anyone else).

The result is that there are some genuine phenomena that are described by the term self-deception, but it is very difficult to furnish

166

a satisfactory explanation of how self-deception can happen. For Freud, this difficulty was resolved by suggesting that the sensitive information was kept in the unconscious, and some intrapsychic censor accomplished self-deception by keeping the conscious self unaware of the guilty knowledge that resided in the unconscious. Unfortunately, modern psychology can no longer easily accept the notion of an unconscious as a kind of mysterious bucket, full of things that belong to the self but are not recognized by the conscious mind. This is not to reject the wisdom of Freud's insights, but only to find his metaphors becoming too clumsy.

The conceptual problem is that there is an innate contradiction in the concept of self-deception, for one cannot be both the (knowing) deceiver and the (unknowing) dupe. Yet to put things that way is probably too black and white to be correct. Human beliefs and opinions often exist among shades of gray—possibilities, probable truths, working assumptions, leaps to conclusions. In this large gray area there is plenty of room for errors and distortions to arise. Self-deception can flourish by capitalizing on these distortions.

Explicit, objective facts allow little room for self-deception. The fact that one is divorced, or has lost one's job, cannot easily be concealed from the self. But where subjective impressions and judgments are concerned, there is more room for distortion—for the subtle shadings that may allow self-deception. Is your marriage extremely happy, or just moderately happy? Did you lose your job because you were incompetent, or was it because they made you a scapegoat and blamed you for things that were not really your fault? Answers to such questions are important *and* relatively immune to objective verification. So although it is hard to deceive oneself about whether one is divorced or not, it is quite possible to deceive oneself about *why* one's marriage had to end—about who started the arguments, whose misdeeds were most fatal, or whether the marriage could have succeeded under other circumstances.

Once we come to see self-deception in terms of shades of gray, then it can be recognized everywhere. Most people consider themselves to be smarter than the average person, and more attractive, and a better driver, and so forth. These small exaggerations of one's own good points are a pervasive feature of how the normal person sees himself or herself (Taylor & Brown, 1988). Indeed, researchers who study self-esteem have begun to recognize that there are relatively few people, at least in modern America, who have genuinely low self-esteem. What researchers had always done was simply collect a large sample of people, measure their self-esteem with a standard questionnaire form, and divide the scores in half, calling the high scores "high self-esteem" and the low scores "low self-esteem." But recent evidence has accumulated to suggest that these below-average scores are actually medium in an absolute sense (see Baumeister, Tice, & Hutton, 1989). The average level of self-esteem is high. Although everyone feels bad about himself or herself occasionally, very few people really hold consistently low opinions of themselves.

One might suppose that there are pockets of low self-esteem among certain disadvantaged segments of the population. After all, social scientists have been expounding theories for decades about how society sends messages of inferiority to blacks, women, and other groups, and so inevitably they must start to believe these messages. But the evidence has accumulated to indicate that such belief is not so inevitable after all. If anything, blacks have slightly higher self-esteem than whites, and women have slightly higher self-esteem than men (Crocker & Major, 1989).

How do people sustain these generally favorable views of themselves? To answer that question, it is necessary to investigate the techniques of self-deception. The self-deceiver's goal is to protect his/her favorable view of self at all costs, and people employ a number of strategies to accomplish this.

A first strategy is to pay attention selectively. This brings us back to the philosophical dilemma of self-deception, for seemingly one must first notice something in order to be careful not to notice it—but if one has already noticed it, then it is too late. To resolve this dilemma, it is only necessary to recall that we are not dealing with absolutes but only with differences of degree. People may notice unpleasant truths but simply not dwell on them. One can pass quickly over the bad news but linger to savor the good news.

Evidence of this strategy emerged from an experiment with a group of students who were carefully selected as having particularly repressive personalities—that is, people particularly inclined toward self-deception. These students took a personality test and then received phony feedback about themselves. By random assignment, some were given favorable, even flattering feedback, whereas others received sharply critical, unfavorable feedback. The researchers secretly timed how long each individual spent studying the bogus feedback. As long as they thought no one but themselves would see the feedback, they showed a clear tendency to avoid the bad news. In other words, the ones who received the harsh criticism spent much less time reading it than the ones who received glowing praise, even though it was exactly the same amount of information (Baumeister & Cairns, 1992).

It is often possible to spot unpleasant things coming and avoid them. One researcher has compared this process to how people handle junk mail (Greenwald, 1988). After all, you don't have to open every envelope and read the contents to know whether you are interested or not. Often, one can recognize junk mail just by looking at the envelope, and so it can be thrown away unopened. In the same way, one can learn to recognize far in advance a person or situation likely to bring embarrassment, threat, criticism, failure, or other bad news, and so one can manage to duck out rather than face the threat.

Paying attention selectively, then, is one means of self-deception. It is not the only one. Another is interpreting events in a biased fashion. As many studies have shown, people tend to take credit for their successes but deny blame for their failures. This is a subtle way of thinking, akin to saying, "Heads I win, tails it's chance." Failure can be blamed on bad luck, mitigating circumstances, unfair bias, or the incompetence of one's mates. Success is readily understood in terms of one's own talents, abilities, and hard work. Self-esteem may in principle be based on a person's balance of successes and failures, but people manage to find reasons for deciding that some of the failures *don't count.*

This pattern of self-serving bias helps explain how most people can continue to think of themselves as above average. On any given exam, for example, half the students perform below the class average, and so in theory just as many people receive bad feedback as good feedback. But those who receive the bad feedback will tend to discount it—blaming a bad night's sleep, unfairness in the test, bad luck in guessing or in having studied the wrong topics, and so forth. But do the students who get the top grades similarly dismiss this news as due to some lucky guesses or in choice of questions, to unfair bias in their favor, or to an especially good night's sleep? Hardly. Instead, they are likely to see the good grade as an accurate recognition of their keen intelligence, thorough knowledge, and diligent preparation.

The self-serving bias also helps explain the surprising fact, noted above, that stigmatized groups often end up with self-esteem levels equal to or higher than that of advantaged groups. A history of bias gives people a ready-made excuse for failure. If one can dismiss one's failures as caused by other people's racism or sexism, one can then base one's self-esteem solely on one's successes, and as a result it can stay strong (see Crocker & Major, 1989). A vivid example of this was provided in 1990 when Marion Barry, the mayor of Washington D.C., was arrested and put on trial for using illegal drugs (among other offenses). In that case, the prosecution had a film of him smoking cocaine in a hotel room with a woman with whom he had had extramarital sex, and in addition there was substantial testimony as to his drug use on other occasions. But instead of accepting the disgrace as an understandable result of his illegal and immoral actions, Barry charged that he was being persecuted simply because he belonged to an ethnic minority group. In his view, his problems did not reflect his own failings but rather the fact that others were biased against him. Likewise, in 1991, when judge Clarence Thomas's confirmation as a Supreme Court justice was nearly ruined by allegations of sexual harassment, Thomas complained that he was being unfairly persecuted because of racism and compared his situation to that of lynching victims, scarcely bothering even to account for the fact that his main accuser was just as black as he was! Such a style of thinking allows people to maintain their self-esteem at a high level, for it dismisses the potential implications of one's failures or misdeeds.

Yet another technique of self-deception involves biased reasoning. When people draw conclusions, they often end up with what they wanted to believe. This pattern can sometimes creates the false impression that people just arbitrarily and peremptorily decide to believe whatever they want to believe. In fact, people try to be objective and often fail to see the biases in their own reasoning. People may know what conclusion they want, but they try to be fair and to construct an argument that would persuade an unbiased observer or judge (Kunda, 1990).

If they try to be fair, how is it that bias creeps in? One decisive factor is hidden in the way people construct arguments. When people are trying to decide whether something is true, they search for evidence that confirms it—rather than for evidence that refutes it. This is a general tendency in human thought, and it poses problems for scientists, troubleshooters, and others concerned with establishing truth. For the self-deceiver, however, it is a handy mechanism.

Suppose, for example, that you are a parent wondering about how bright your child is. You are likely to have a preferred conclusion—most parents want to think their child is unusually intelligent. But you don't just leap to that desired conclusion without evidence. You try to evaluate the evidence, by reviewing things your child has done or said. In reviewing it, however, you are likely to search for the especially bright things your child has said or done, which support what you want to believe. If, instead, you tried to think of the especially stupid and inept moments in your child's past, you might be led to a different conclusion. But by focusing on the positive signs, one can build a logical case for the desired conclusion.

When one has done something wrong and potentially objection-able, another group of self-deceptive strategies comes into play. In our research, we have compared how victims and offenders describe events, and offenders seem to have several ways of minimizing their guilt. One is to downplay the consequences; whereas victims tend to perceive substantial harm and other negative consequences, offenders tend to minimize the damage. Another, more interesting strategy is to isolate the incident conceptually, in a sense burying it in the past. In examining the time structure of people's narratives, a striking difference emerged. Victims wrote of events leading up to the offense, of the event itself, and of its lasting consequences and implications, often spanning years and extending up to the present and even the future. In contrast, offenders tended to describe only the event itself, as if cut off from past and future. In some cases they explicitly said it was an isolated incident unrelated to prior or subsequent events. Thus, they managed to reduce any feelings of guilt or obligation by treating the incident as something that was over and done and had no relation to the rest of their lives (Baumeister, Stillwell, & Wotman, 1991).

History furnishes some vivid illustrations of this "isolation" mode of self-deception, by which victims and offenders end up with radically different views of past transgressions. Anyone who has lived in both the northern and the southern parts of the United States knows how radically they differ in views about the Civil War. To northerners, the Civil War is ancient history, something their forefathers went through in order to help rid the nation of the evil institution of slavery and preserve the constitutional union. Everything soon went back to normal, and apart from a few beneficial effects such as the freeing of the slaves, northerners probably think that very little about today's America is a direct result of that war. In contrast, the southerners still nurse feelings of anger and humiliation at the cruel destruction of their culture and way of life by northerners bent on imposing their will with military power. Southerners do not accept the view that the war was all about slavery, and they see many of today's social problems, especially in the south, as a result of the war.

If that example is not enough, one can examine the even more extreme case of the Crusades. Western histories of the Crusades (e.g., Runciman, 1951–1954) treat those long-forgotten events in the context of medieval history, religious idealism, the need to protect European pilgrims to the Holy Land, and curiosities of military strategies and methods. They acknowledge that certain excesses and atrocities occurred (e.g., burning villages to the ground, massacring innocent civilians and even hostages, roasting and eating Moslem babies) but these are deplored as the unfortunate sort of thing that occurred back then, certainly with no relation to Westerners of today. The consequences of the Crusades are described in terms of increased trade, cultural exchange, and other positive outcomes, most of which have in turn been long absorbed into the stream of history and swamped by other events. Few would see direct relevance of the Crusades to today's world. In contrast, a recent history of the Crusades from the Arab perspective (Maalouf, 1987) concluded forcefully that today's Moslems and Arabs have vivid memories of the Crusades and consider those events quite relevant to today's issues. From the Moslem view, the Arabs were simply minding their own business when the European Christians repeatedly attacked without provocation, behaving in a generally savage and uncivilized fashion, breaking rules of war and honor, and committing unspeakable atrocities. The consequences were neither positive nor temporary; rather, the flowering of Moslem Arab culture was brought to an end and replaced by a period of brutality and stagnation. All of this, according to Maalouf, still forms the foundation of how today's Moslem Arabs perceive Westerners and Christians. Maalouf says that current Arab practices and policies, including the oil embargoes and the support for terrorism, can only be understood in terms of the lasting distrust of the Westerners based on the Moslems' sense of victimization. They do not see any reason to believe that modern Europeans and Americans are fundamentally any better than the liars, thieves, rapists, and killers who wrought such havoc in their land during the Crusades.

Examples could be enumerated endlessly. It would be rash to propose that only the offenders engage in self-deception; for all we know, victims too can distort memories to exaggerate them, just as offenders minimize them. You, the reader, are probably descended from Europeans, yet probably you do not feel personally guilty over the Crusades and may in fact think it excessive for the Arabs to bear a grudge over so many centuries. My point is simply that offenders seek to minimize negative consequences and bury transgressions in the past, and that such styles of thinking *may* be used for purposes of self-deception. Isolating an event, temporally and conceptually, steadily diminishes its meaning.

Atrocity, war, and death form important contexts for self-deception, but people fool themselves in love too. Such patterns have been documented in our recent research on unrequited love (Baumeister & Wotman, 1992). Unrequited love forms a common context for self-deception. In our research, one out of every five broken-hearted lovers spontaneously said that he or she had engaged in self-deception during the episode, and undoubtedly the actual rate of self-deception is significantly higher than that. (Indeed, seen from the other side self-deception was certainly more prevalent; two out of every five rejectors spontaneously described their admirers as having engaged in self-deception!) Love brings a sense of optimism and hope, and thousands of novels, movies, and other stories have reiterated the theme that initial rejection or indifference can be overcome if the would-be lover persists. That does seem to be how people act. As one man wrote of his experience, "There were certainly enough cues as to her lack of attraction for me, but I was too preoccupied to notice. At that point, my feelings were of the stereotype, 'I'm so happy that I'm with her, I couldn't care less about anything.' " Thus, he was in love with her, and he simply ignored the discouraging signs about her lack of reciprocal interest in him.

A further reason for self-deception among aspiring lovers is that rejection is a threat to one's self-esteem. At the core of mating, after all, is equity; people marry people who are roughly equal to themselves in various ways. Romantic rejection thus carries an implicit and often well-founded message that "You are simply not good enough for me." People are reluctant to accept that message, and in the long run it proved one of the hardest things for people to accept about being rejected. Likewise, people find it humiliating to accept that the time they spent with people they loved was casual or trivial to these others. For example, one woman in our study described an experience in which she gave her virginity to a fellow she loved but who, it turned out, never cared much about her and regarded her merely as a casual sexual fling or conquest. It was hard enough to accept his rejection of her in the end, but it was even harder for her to face the fact that he had never loved her. "Of course, I was blind to this fact for a long time because I refused to admit that I slept with someone who cared less [for me than I cared for him]." Her inclusion of the phrase "of course" is revealing: She suggested that it is inevitable that she would be reluctant to face the heartbreaking, humiliating truth.

During the phase of self-deception, aspiring lovers grasp desperately for any means of explaining away the discouraging signs they receive from the other. If she is cold and distant, perhaps she is just in a bad mood. If he says straight out that he does not love you, perhaps he is just denying his true feelings. All of this is complicated by the rejector's inner struggles with guilt and awkwardness and simple reluctance to inflict pain on someone. Few rejectors come right out and say, "I don't think you are good enough for me" or "I find you ugly, boring, and stupid." Instead, they try to soften the blow with diplomatic or kind words that unfortunately blunt the message and make it ambiguous. They say, "You are a wonderful person and I know someday you will make someone very happy, and I have really enjoyed being with you and want to remain close friends, but I just do not feel I want a romantic relationship with you right now." After such a speech, the rejector thinks the matter is over and done, the message delivered. But the aspiring lover has heard only a mixed message: This person thinks I am wonderful, thinks I will make a good mate, isn't quite ready to make a commitment to me now, but wants to keep a close relationship with me. Often the rejector is shocked and resentful when the romantic attentions and advances continue.

In summary, while it may be true that no one can both know and not know the same thing at the same time, there is still room for self-deception. The lies one tells to oneself are rarely whoppers. Instead, they are fibs, exaggerations, selective omissions, best-case scenarios, and other distortions. Self-deception resembles propaganda rather than perjury. When objective evidence is solid, self-deception tends to vanish, for having seen the black one cannot usually convince oneself that it was indeed white. But when the facts come in shifting shades of gray there is ample room for fooling oneself about their average degree of whiteness.

LYING TO SELF AND OTHERS

We now turn to consider the relationship between lying to oneself and lying to others. At first blush, there is little necessary relationship between the two. You can lie to others while clearly knowing the truth yourself. On the other hand, it is hard to lie to yourself while telling the truth to others. They may recognize the truth even if you do not, but if you recognize the truth well enough to tell them directly, your chances for succeeding at self-deception are slim.

Other people thus put some limits on one's latitude for self-deception. If they enter the picture at all, then one has to lie to them too—or else give up lying to oneself.

This has serious ramifications for self-deception. For one thing, the self may be an unusually sympathetic audience, but other people are not likely to be so sympathetic. As we saw in the previous section, people lie to themselves by focusing on evidence for what they want to believe and conveniently overlooking contrary signals. But you cannot necessarily trust other people to overlook those contrary signals too. As a result, some self-deceptive strategies that succeed in the privacy of one's own mind may become useless when other people are involved.

Earlier, I described an experiment in which people passed over critical feedback quickly, preferring to tune out and ignore it, but spent much longer periods of time reading complimentary, favorable feedback (Baumeister & Cairns, 1992). That self-deceptive strategy was what people preferred—as long as people thought the feedback was completely confidential. Other participants in that same study, however, were told that their personality evaluation was also being shown to someone else whom they expected to meet in a few minutes. That changed everything. It was no longer enough to simply ignore the criticism, for it would not go away just by pretending it was not there. You might ignore it, but you could not expect someone else to ignore it too. The pattern of skipping quickly through the criticism disappeared when people were told that someone else had access to that information. Indeed, these people spent longer reading the criticism than reading the praise! It is very important to know how one is viewed by someone else, and one has to be especially careful when others know bad things about you.

Two factors enter into the process when information is public. First, the information gains *social reality* (Wicklund & Gollwitzer, 1982). You cannot make it disappear simply by ignoring it. It exists outside your mind, and that confers some reality on it that takes it out of your exclusive control. Second, you may have to interact with these other people, and so you need to anticipate how they will regard you and treat you.

As a result, some self-deceptive strategies must be abandoned when other people become involved. True, a sympathetic audience—such as a staunchly supportive and loyal mate—may simply buttress your self-deceptions by telling you what you want to hear and reaffirming your preferred views (see Swann & Predmore, 1985). This is one of the dangers of power, of course, for sycophantic underlings and yes-men can encourage the leader's illusions. Most of the time, however, other people represent a likely or actual challenge to one's illusions and preferred beliefs. Other people thus serve as a valuable check on self-deception.

But that is only half the picture. Just as others' disbelief can undermine one's own belief, so can their positive belief support one's preferred view. In other words, if you can manage to convince others, that is a big help toward convincing yourself.

Child abusers form a compelling, if sinister, example of the manipulation of others in the service of self-deception. Research by Korbin (1987a, 1987b, 1989) examined women who had eventually killed their children; the deaths were typically preceded by years of escalating mistreatment. These women had hurt their children many times, often requiring medical attention. Such injuries cannot of course be ignored.

Consider the self-deception project of the child abuser. No woman wants to consider herself an unfit mother or as a person who violently harms her own helpless, innocent babies. If she does cause them harm, her view of herself as a good mother is in jeopardy, and so she must lie to herself that the child's injury is an isolated event, an accident—not a reflection of the kind of mother she is.

If the child is simply bruised, the mother can perhaps rationalize the event as an accident or as an unfortunate consequence of something that was really the child's fault. But injury requires medical attention, which means bringing other people in, and so the first self-deceptive strategy (i.e., ignoring it) is not viable. In Korbin's account, the women converted the encounter with the physicians into a test of the truth. Like many Americans, they tended to regard physicians as godlike figures whose judgment carried great weight and finality. Would the physician condemn them as bad mothers?

What typically happened was that the physician focused his or her attention on the injury to the child and did not ask much about how it had happened, perhaps accepting some casual explanation offered by the mother. Korbin emphasizes the relief that the woman typically felt. She had not concealed her child's injury but had in fact taken it to the clinic for all the world to see, and yet she had come through it all without being pronounced a bad mother. To the mother, the physician's lack of reaction or judgment was converted into an affirmation of her fitness as a mother. In her own mind, she transformed the physician into an accomplice of her lies to herself.

Furthermore, the abusive mother was typically shrewd enough to bias this test in her favor. She might describe the injury by saying her child fell down the stairs, leaving out the part about how she had pushed the child to cause the fall. (Perhaps she was willing to disclose that if asked, but the question never came—which seemed to prove that it was not important.) More important, the next time something similar happened, she would take the child to a different hospital or clinic, where a different physician would see the child. In her view, this might provide that much more support for her status as a good mother, for now several different physicians had seen the child's injuries but no one had reproached or accused her of being a bad mother. Overlooked in this reasoning, of course, is the fact that the very multiplicity of doctors prevented any one of them from seeing the pattern of repeated injuries. A physician is probably always reluctant to make an accusation of child abuse, especially from a single incident, and so one would only become suspicious—or at least, would only become overtly accusatory—after repeated injuries. No physician was given the chance to see the pattern, and so no accusations were forthcoming. But the woman did not have to think through all those complexities or subtleties. She could simply dwell on the fact that she had taken the child to many doctors and none of them had ever said anything to her. In short, she manipulated the circumstances and the other people to aid her lies to self. Apparently the project worked for many of them, for they were able to sustain this view of themselves as a good mother, until the day the child died.

In summary, other people are both a problem and an opportunity for the self-deceiver. A person who wants to believe something finds it easier to believe if others can be induced to believe it, or even just to go along with it. Lying to others can thus be a means of lying to oneself. On the other hand, a carefully woven network of self-deceptions can be rudely disrupted if other people fail to validate it or point out its fallacies. Self-deception is thus easiest to accomplish in the privacy of one's own mind. But if other people become involved, it becomes urgently necessary to convince them as well.

EFFECTS OF SELF-DECEPTION

It may be easy to make a moral judgment about self-deception, but to judge its psychological consequences one must first look carefully at its costs and benefits. There is evidence of both.

Conventional wisdom has condemned self-deception as an unhealthy lack of contact with reality. The view of mental health and adjustment as requiring accurate perception of self and world has recently received some severe shocks, however. After years of assuming that depressed people suffered from a distorted view of things, psychologists were surprised when evidence began to emerge that depressed people tend to see events more accurately than non-depressed people (Alloy & Abramson, 1979). A broad review by Taylor and Brown (1988) has asserted that seeing the world (including oneself) in a favorably distorted fashion is an integral part of healthy adjustment. In other words, regular doses of self-deception are good for you.

Consider some of the benefits of these "positive illusions" (Taylor & Brown, 1988; Taylor, 1989). In the first place, it is emotionally pleasant to overestimate one's abilities, to be optimistic, and to believe one is generally in control of events. There is little doubt about this. After all, why would people lie to themselves at all, if not for the sake of feeling better? The scholar and psychotherapist C.R. Snyder recalls trying to convince one of his patients to face the truth about some matter, and the patient grumbled, "What's so great about reality, anyway?" If we can successfully persuade ourselves of our marvelous talents and excellent prospects, we are likely to feel considerably happier than if we force ourselves to keep a sober outlook illuminated only by the harsh light of reality.

Moreover, it may be necessary to deceive oneself in order to have a realistic chance at some of life's peak experiences. At the extreme, one may question whether anyone would attain life's greatest human fulfillments, such as major career success, passionate love, or religious salvation, without being helped along by some illusions. Grand ambition, romantic passion, and religious faith all require some heavy doses of faith and optimism beyond what is strictly warranted by the facts.

A particularly important process here is the *self-fulfilling prophecy*. Sometimes believing that something is true helps make it come true. The most familiar indication of this is the simple effect of confidence on performance. Expecting to succeed will often actually help you succeed (Feather, 1966, 1968, 1969; also Baumeister, Hamilton, & Tice, 1985). By the same token, expecting to fail will sometimes make failure more likely. There is thus a practical advantage of lying to yourself. By exaggerating your assessment of your chances of success, you can actually improve those chances. This is a lesson that lies close to America's heart, and it is drummed into the collective mind from early childhood (*The Little Engine That Could*) to adulthood (as in the "can-do" attitude, or the necessity of avoiding "negative thinking").

Of course, sometimes our optimism turns out to be misplaced, and we are confronted with misfortunes. Even then, however, it is apparently beneficial to engage in self-deception. Recovering from trauma often involves rebuilding one's sense that the world is a safe place and one is in control of one's fate (Janoff-Bulman, 1985, 1989; Taylor, 1983). Sometimes coping requires convincing oneself of quite dubious propositions. For example, Taylor (1983, 1989) found that many cancer victims succeeded in convincing themselves that they could prevent the cancer from coming back or from spreading. The methods that held their faith, ranging from changing one's diet to changing one's spouse, had little or no justification in medical knowledge, but the cancer victims were better off (measured in terms of coping and adjustment) as long as they held that faith.

Thus, self-deception has its advantages. But there are costs as well. Sometimes being out of touch with reality can be dangerous. For one thing, confidence is not always enough, and boasts can look foolish in retrospect. In the days leading up to the 1988 Super Bowl, the television announcers marveled at the superb confidence shown by the Denver team leader and quarterback John Elway. They agreed that he was completely ready for the game and was infusing his entire team with an unshakable belief in their coming victory. Instead of the expected triumph, however, Denver suffered a thorough and humiliating defeat. Indeed, the Washington team set several Super Bowl records at Denver's expense. Two years later, a Denver poll found a majority of local fans hoping their team would lose early in the playoffs rather than make it back to the Super Bowl and face a repeat of that humiliation.

Confidence may often benefit performances, but it can mislead and confound decision processes. Overconfidence can cloud one's judgment and lead people to take on projects or make commitments at which they have little chance of success. Thus, the real costs of self-deception may be found in bad or costly decisions.

History furnishes numerous examples of the perils of overconfidence. From Napoleon's invasion of Russia to America's misadventure in Vietnam, there are ample demonstrations that overestimating one's military might and invincibility periodically leads to disaster. The medieval Crusades were spurred by the faith that God would guarantee Christian victory over heathens and infidels, a faith that was sadly disappointed in the end. The Children's Crusade in particular was motivated by the firm belief that God would protect the innocents and even part the Mediterranean Sea in order for them to march across to Jerusalem. Instead, most of the participants died or were sold into slavery (Cohn, 1970; see also Runciman, 1951–1954).

The battlefield is not the only place where history reveals the perils of overconfidence. In the 1970s, the Khmer Rouge succeeded militarily in conquering Cambodia. After their victory, their leaders set about instituting their plan to make Cambodia into a self-sufficient agricultural nation. The Cambodian economy had only been viable on the basis of foreign aid, which the Khmer Rouge now refused to accept; the belief that city dwellers could be converted overnight into successful rice farmers was tragically absurd; the beaver-style dams built by peasants, without the anti-flooding safeguards favored by the despised foreign-educated engineers, were disastrous; and so forth. The outcome was widespread starvation, economic failure, and an escalating search for scapegoats that ended in terrorist purges and mass murder (Becker, 1986).

The dangers of overconfidence are also apparent at the individual level. One realm where self-deception can be harmful, even fatal, is sexual behavior. Many people know that unprotected sexual intercourse can result in pregnancy and venereal disease, yet they continue to think that "It can't happen to me" and fail to take precautions. Researchers have dubbed this the "illusion of unique invulnerability" because the individual knows that these consequences happen to others but assumes that such things will not happen to himself or herself (Burger & Burns, 1988). As the recent AIDS epidemic spread, many people refused to believe in the dangers and continued their unsafe practices. This included both the gay community, which sometimes fought to sustain bathhouses and other places where large-scale promiscuity spread disease rapidly, and the blood bank industry which long refused to acknowledge the possibility that contaminated blood samples could be fatal to helpless, unsuspecting people receiving transfusions. Chronicler Randy Shilts (1987) described America's response to AIDS in 1983 as "denial on all fronts, leading to stupid mistakes that would costs thousands of lives in the short term and tens of thousands in the long term" (p. 224).

Recent laboratory research has even suggested that high self-esteem can lead to bad judgment and costly mistakes. Overconfident people tend to take on too much or set goals too high for themselves, especially when their self-esteem is challenged. As a result, they may often experience severe failure (Baumeister, Heatherton, & Tice, in press). Investing your effort in pursuing a career that is beyond your abilities will lead eventually to failure, just as putting your money into a house or other purchase that is beyond your means will lead to an ongoing struggle to make the payments and, eventually, to repossession and severe financial loss. People with high self-esteem are prone to overestimate their performance capabilities, and these errors can cause them to get in over their heads, often with disastrous results. Indeed, recent evidence indicates that people with high self-esteem are more likely than others to not wear helmets while riding motorcycles! (Pelham & Taylor, 1991).

CONCLUSION

Self-deception is here to stay. For one thing, it appears to have benefits, as already noted: It helps people feel good, recover from trauma, sustain the confidence for tackling difficult problems and succeeding, and so forth. Moreover, self-deception is big business in America. Advertisers encourage people to believe that purchasing various products will make them attractive, sexy, glamorous, rich, and so forth. Pop psychologists write best-selling books exhorting people to think more positively about themselves (see Huber, 1987, for a long-term perspective on this aspect of American thought). The diet industry makes immense sums of money by convincing people that they can become slim, despite accumulating evidence that nearly all the weight lost on diets is regained (see Polivy & Herman, 1983).

There are two ways to live with self-deception and avoid disaster. One is to confine oneself to telling only little white lies to oneself. There is some evidence that people do indeed keep their illusions and self-deceptions down to a relatively small size. People may exaggerate their abilities, virtues, and prospects slightly, but they avoid drastic exaggerations (Baumeister, 1989). They remain within this optimal margin of illusion—neither seeing things too accurately and realistically, nor allowing their distortions to become too large. That way, they can enjoy the emotional benefits of these illusions without suffering the practical consequences of clouded judgment.

The other way is to shift back and forth between realism and self-deception. This is not necessarily easy to do, but there is some evidence that people can manage it sometimes (Gollwitzer & Kinney, 1989). All that is necessary is to have two habitual frames of mind, one suitable for making judgments and decisions, the other suitable for action and performance. When judgment and decision are required, the mind becomes realistic and tries to proceed with accurate assessments of self and world. When the decision is completed and it is time for action, the person shifts into a confident, optimistic attitude, characterized by favorably distorted views. It is a delicate balancing act, but it can be done to some extent.

It would be reckless to condemn all self-deception as bad or harmful, and it would be absurd to hope that it can eventually be eliminated. Certain self-deceptive patterns are widespread and deeply ingrained, and for good reason. After all, sometimes people do benefit from having some confidence, optimism, or faith that goes beyond what reality warrants. Perhaps the optimum is to learn to keep self-deception within safe bounds and thus to enable it to learn to work for us, rather than against us. Perhaps we can all learn to to manage our self-deceptive tendencies effectively and channel them to our long-term advantage. Perhaps, in short, we can learn to make self-deception into our trusted servant. But perhaps that optimistic hope is itself a sign that we are just fooling ourselves.

References

Alloy, L. B., & Abramson, L. (1979). Judgment of contingency in depressed and nondepressed students: Sadder but wiser? *Journal of Experimental Psychology: General, 108*, 441–485.

Baumeister, R. F. (1989). The optimal margin of illusion. *Journal of Social and Clinical Psychology*,8, 176–189.

Baumeister, R. F., & Cairns, K. J. (1992). Repression and self-presentation: When audiences interfere with self-deceptive strategies. *Journal of Personality and Social Psychology, 62*, 851–862.

Baumeister, R. F., Hamilton, J. C., & Tice, D. M. (1985). Public versus private expectancy of success: Confidence booster or performance pressure? *Journal of Personality and Social Psychology, 48*, 1447–1457.

Baumeister, R. F., Heatherton, T. F., & Tice, D. M. (in press). When ego threats lead to self-regulation failure: Negative consequences of high self-esteem. *Journal of Personality and Social Psychology*.

Baumeister, R. F., Stillwell, A., & Wotman, S. R. (1990). Victim and perpetrator accounts of interpersonal conflict: Autobiographical narratives about anger. *Journal of Personality and Social Psychology, 59*, 994–1005.

Baumeister, R. F., Tice, D. M., & Hutton, D. G. (1989). Self-presentational motivations and personality differences in self-esteem. *Journal of Personality, 57*, 547–579.

Baumeister, R. F., & Wotman, S. R. (1992). *Breaking hearts: The two sides of unrequited love*. New York: Guilford Press.

Becker, E. (1986). *When the war was over*. New York: Simon & Schuster.

Burger, J. M., & Burns, L. (1988). The illusion of unique invulnerability and the use of effective contraception. *Personality and Social Psychology Bulletin, 14*. 264–270.

Cohn, N. (1970). *The pursuit of the millenium: Revolutionary millenarians and mystical anarchists of the Middle Ages*. New York: Oxford University Press.

Crocker, J., & Major, B. (1989). Social stigma and self-esteem: The self-protective properties of stigma. *Psychological Review, 96*, 608–630.

Feather, N. T. (1966). Effects of prior success and failure on expectations of success and subsequent performance. *Journal of Personality and Social Psychology, 3*, 287–298.

Feather, N. T. (1968). Change in confidence following success or failure as a predictor of subsequent performance. *Journal of Personality and Social Psychology, 13*, 129–144.

Feather, N. T. (1969). Attribution of responsibility and valence of success and failure in relation to initial confidence and task performance. *Journal of Personality and Social Psychology, 13*, 129–144.

Gollwitzer, P. M., & Kinney, R. F. (1989). Effects of deliberative and implemental mind-sets on illusion of control. *Journal of Personality and Social Psychology, 56*, 531–542.

Greenwald, A. G. (1988). Self-knowledge and self-deception. In J. B. Lockard & D. Paulhus (Eds.), *Self-deception: An adaptive mechanism?* (pp. 113–131). Englewood Cliffs, NJ: Prentice-Hall.

Huber, R. M. (1987). *The American idea of success*. Wainscott, NY: Pushcart Press. Originally published in 1971 by McGraw-Hill.

Janoff-Bulman, R. (1985). The aftermath of victimization: Rebuilding shattered assumptions. In C. R. Figley (Ed.), *Trauma and its wake* (pp. 15–35). New York: Brunner/Mazel.

Janoff-Bulman, R. (1989). Assumptive worlds and the stress of traumatic events: Applications of the schema construct. *Social Cognition, 7,* 113–136.

Korbin, J. (1987a: July). *Fatal child maltreatment.* Paper presented at the Third National Family Violence Research Conference, Durham NH.

Korbin, J. (1987b). Incarcerated mothers' perceptions and interpretations of their fatally maltreated children. *Child Abuse & Neglect, 11,* 397–407.

Korbin, J. (1989). Fatal maltreatment by mothers: A proposed framework. *Child Abuse & Neglect, 13,* 481–489.

Kunda, Z. (1990). The case for motivated reasoning. *Psychological Bulletin, 108,* 480–498.

Maalouf, A. (1987). *The Crusades through Arab eyes* (J. Rothschild, trans.). New York: Schocken.

Pelham, B. W., & Taylor, S. E. (1991). *On the limits of illusions: Exploring the costs and hazards of high self-regard.* Unpublished manuscript, University of California at Los Angeles.

Polivy, J., & Herman, C. P. (1983). *Breaking the diet habit: The natural weight alternative.* New York: Basic Books.

Runciman, S. (1951–1954). *A history of the Crusades* (3 vols.). Cambridge, England: Cambridge University Press.

Russell, F. H. (1975). *The just war in the Middle Ages.* Cambridge, England: Cambridge University Press.

Sackeim, H. A., & Gur, R. C. (1979). Self-deception, other-deception, and self-reported psychopathology. *Journal of Consulting and Clinical Psychology, 47,* 213–215.

Sartre, J.-P. (1953) *The existential psychoanalysis.* (H. E. Barnes, trans.) New York: Philosophical Library.

Shilts, R. (1987). *And the band played on: Politics, people, and the AIDS epidemic.* New York: Viking Penguin.

Swann, W. B., & Predmore, S. (1985). Intimates as agents of social support: Sources of consolation or despair? *Journal of Personality and Social Psychology, 49,* 1609–1617.

Taylor, S. E. (1983). Adjustment to threatening events: A theory of cognitive adaptation. *American Psychologist, 38,* 1161–1173.

Taylor, S. E. (1989). *Positive illusions: Creative self-deception and the healthy mind.* New York: Basic Books.

Taylor, S. E., & Brown, J. D. (1988). Illusion and well-being: A social psychological perspective on mental health. *Psychological Bulletin, 103,* 193–210.

Wicklund, R. A., & Gollwitzer, P. M. (1982). *Symbolic self-completion.* Hillsdale, NJ: Erlbaum.

9
Lies That Fail

PAUL EKMAN
MARK G. FRANK

Lies fail for many reasons. Some of these reasons have to do with the circumstances surrounding the lie, and not with the liar's behavior. For example, a confidant may betray a lie; or, private information made public can expose a liar's claims as false. These reasons do not concern us in this chapter. What concerns us are those mistakes made during the act of lying, mistakes liars make despite themselves; in other words, lies that fail because of the liars' behaviors. Deception clues or leakage may be shown in a change in the expression on the face, a movement of the body, an inflection to the voice, a swallowing in the throat, a very deep or shallow breath, long pauses between words, a slip of the tongue, a microfacial expression, or a gestural slip.

There are two basic reasons why lies fail—one that involves thinking, and one that involves emotions. Lies fail due to a failure of the liar to prepare his or her line, or due to the interference of emotions. These reasons have different implications for the potential behavioral clues that betray a lie.

LIES BETRAYED BY THINKING CLUES

Liars do not always anticipate when they will need to lie. There is not always time to prepare the line to be taken, to rehearse and memorize it. Even when there has been ample advance notice, and a false line has been carefully devised, the liar may not be clever enough to anticipate all the questions that may be asked, and to have thought through what his answers must be. Even cleverness may not be enough, for unseen changes in circumstances can betray an otherwise effective line. And, even when a liar is not forced by circumstances to change lines, some liars have trouble recalling the line they have previously committed themselves to, so that new questions cannot be consistently answered quickly.

Any of these failures—in anticipating when it will be necessary to lie, in inventing a line which is adequate to changing circumstances, in remembering the line one has adopted—produce easily spotted clues to deceit. What the person says is either internally inconsistent, or at odds with other incontrovertible facts, known at the time or later revealed. Such obvious clues to deceit are not always as reliable and straightforward as they seem. Too smooth a line may be the sign of a well rehearsed con man. To make matters worse, some con men knowing this purposely make slight mistakes in order not to seem too smooth! This was the case with Clifford Irving, who claimed he was authorized by Howard Hughes to write Hughes' biography. While on trial, Irving deliberately contradicted himself (albeit minor contradictions) because he knew that only liars tell perfectly planned accounts. The psychological evidence supports Irving's notion that planned responses are judged as more deceptive than unplanned ones (DePaulo, Lanier, & Davis, 1983). However, we believe in general that people who fabricate without having prepared their line are more likely to make blatant contradictions, to give evasive and indirect accounts—all of which will ultimately betray their lies.

Lack of preparation or a failure to remember the line one has adopted may produce clues to deceit in *how* a line is spoken, even when there are no inconsistencies in *what* is said. The need to think about each word before it is spoken—weighing possibilities, searching for a word or idea—may be obvious in pauses during speech, speech disfluencies, flattened voice intonation, gaze aversion, or more subtly in a tightening of the lower eyelid or eye brow, certain changes in gesture, and a decrease in the use of the hands to illustrate speech (illustrators—Ekman & Friesen, 1969). Not that carefully considering each word before it is spoken is always a sign of deceit, but in some circumstances it is—particularly in contexts in which responses should be known without thought.

LYING ABOUT FEELINGS

A failure to think ahead, plan fully, and rehearse the false line is only one of the reasons why mistakes are made when lying, which then furnish clues to the deceit. Mistakes are also made because of difficulty in concealing or falsely portraying emotion. Not every lie involves emotions, but those that do cause special problems for the liar. An attempt to conceal an emotion at the moment it is felt could be betrayed in words, but except for a slip of the tongue, it usually is not. Unless there is a wish to confess what is felt, the liar does not have to put into words the feelings being concealed. One has less choice in concealing a facial expression, or rapid breathing, or a tightening in the voice.

When emotions are aroused changes occur automatically without choice or deliberation. These changes begin in a split second; this is a fundamental characteristic of emotional experience (Fridja, 1986). People do not actively decide to feel an emotion; instead, they usually experience emotions as happening to them. Negative emotions, such as fear, anger, or sadness, may occur despite either efforts to avoid them (Swann, Griffin, Predmore, & Gaines, 1987), or efforts to hide them (Ekman, Friesen, & O'Sullivan, 1988).

These are what we will call "reliable" behavioral signs of emotion, reliable in the sense that few people can mimic them at all or correctly. Narrowing the red margins of the lips in anger is an example of such a reliable sign of anger, typically missing when anger is feigned, because most people can not voluntarily make that movement. Likewise, when people experience enjoyment they not only move their lip corners upward and back (in a prototypical smile), but they also show a simultaneous contraction of the muscles that surround the eye socket (which raises the cheek, lowers the brow, and creates a "crows feet" appearance). This eye muscle contraction is typically missing from the smile when enjoyment is feigned or not felt (Davidson, Ekman, Saron, Senulius, & Friesen, 1991; Ekman, Davidson, & Friesen, 1991; Frank, Ekman, & Friesen, 1991). And, as in the case of the involuntary movement of the red margins of the lips in anger, most people cannot voluntarily make this eye muscle movement when they are not truly feeling enjoyment (Hager & Ekman, 1985).

Falsifying an experienced emotion is more difficult when one is also attempting to conceal another emotion. Trying to look angry is not easy, but if fear is felt when the person tries to look angry, conflicting forces occur. One set of impulses, arising from fear, pulls in one direction, while the deliberate attempt to appear angry pulls in the other direction. For example, the brows are involuntarily pulled upward and together in fear, but to falsify anger the person must pull them down (Ekman & Friesen, 1975). Often the signs of this internal struggle between the felt and the false emotion betray the deceit (Ekman, Friesen, & O'Sullivan, 1988).

Usually, lies about emotions involve more than just fabricating an emotion which is not felt. They also require concealing an emotion which is being experienced. Concealment often goes hand in hand with fabrication. The liar feigns emotion to mask signs of the emotion to be concealed. Such concealment attempts may be betrayed in either of two ways: (1) some signs of the concealed emotion may escape efforts to inhibit or mask it, providing what Ekman and Friesen (1969) termed *leakage*; or (2) what they called a *deception clue* does not leak the concealed emotion but betrays the likelihood that a lie is being perpetrated. Deception clues occur when only a fragment leaks which is not decipherable, but which does not jibe with the verbal line being maintained by the liar, or when the very effort of having to conceal produces alterations in behavior, and those behavioral alterations do not fit the liar's line.

FEELINGS ABOUT LYING

Not all deceits involve concealing or falsifying emotions. The embezzler conceals that she is stealing money. The plagiarizer conceals that he has taken the words of another and pretends they are his own. The vain middle-aged man conceals his real age, dying his gray hair and claiming he is seven years younger than he is. Yet even when the lie is about something other than emotion, emotions may become involved. The vain man might be embarrassed about his vanity. To succeed in his deceit he must conceal not only his age but his embarrassment as well. The plagiarizer might feel contempt toward those he misleads. He would thus have to conceal not only the source of his work and pretend an ability that is not his, but also conceal his contempt. The embezzler might feel surprise when someone else is accused of her crime. She would have to conceal her surprise or at least conceal the reason why she is surprised.

Thus, emotions often become involved in lies that were not undertaken for the purpose of concealing emotions. Once involved, the emotions must be concealed if the lie is not to be betrayed. Any emotion may be the culprit, but three emotions are so often intertwined with deceit to merit separate explanation: fear of being caught, guilt about lying, and delight in having duped someone.

Fear of Being Caught

In its milder forms, fear of being caught is not disruptive and may even help the deceiver to avoid mistakes by maintaining alertness. Moderate levels of fear can produce behavioral signs that are noticeable by the skilled lie catcher, and high levels of fear produce just what the liar dreads, namely, evidence of his or her fear or apprehension. The research literature on deception detection (DePaulo, Lanier, & Davis, 1983; DePaulo, Stone, & Lassiter, 1985; Zuckerman & Driver, 1985) suggests that the behavior of highly motivated liars is different from that of less motivated ones. In other words, the behavior of liars who fear being caught is different from the behaviors of liars who do not fear being caught.

Many factors influence how the fear of being caught in a lie (or, *detection apprehension*) will be felt. The first determinant to consider is the liar's beliefs about his target's skill as a lie catcher. If the target (i.e., the person being lied to) is known to be gullible, there usually will not be much detection apprehension. On the other hand, a target known to be tough to fool, who has a reputation as an expert lie catcher, will increase the detection apprehension.

The second determinant of detection apprehension is the liar's amount of practice and previous success in lying. A job applicant who has lied about qualifications successfully in the past should not be overly concerned about an additional deception. Practice in deceit enables the liar to anticipate problems. Success in deceit gives confidence and thus reduces the fear of being caught.

The third determinant of detection apprehension is fear of punishment. The fear of being caught can be reduced if the target suggests that the punishment may be less if the liar confesses. Although they usually cannot offer total amnesty, targets may also offer a psychological amnesty, hoping to induce a confession by implying that the liar need not feel ashamed nor even responsible for committing the crime. A target may sympathetically suggest that the acts are understandable and might have been committed by anyone in the same situation. Another variation might be to offer the target a face-saving explanation of the motive for the behavior in which the lie was designed to conceal.

A fourth factor influencing fear of being caught is the personality of the liar. While some people find it easy to lie, others find it difficult to lie; certainly more is known about the former group than the latter (Hood, 1982). One group, called *natural liars* (Ekman, 1985), lie easily and with great success—even though they do not differ from other people on their scores on objective personality tests (Ekman, Friesen, & Scherer, 1976). Natural liars are people who have been getting away with lies since childhood, fooling their parents, teachers, and friends when they wanted to. This instills a sense of confidence in their abilities to deceive such that they have no detection apprehension when they lie. Although this sounds as if natural liars are like psychopaths, they are not; unlike natural liars, psychopaths show poor judgment, no remorse or shame, superficial charm, antisocial behavior without apparent compunction, and pathological egocentricity and incapacity for love (Hare, 1970).

Such natural liars may need to have two very different skills—the skill needed to plan a deceptive strategy, and the skill needed to mislead a target in a face-to-face meeting. A liar might have both skills, but presumably one could excel at one skill and not the other. Regretably, there has been little study of the characteristics of successful deceivers; no research has asked whether the personality characteristics of successful deceivers differ depending on the arena in which the deceit is practiced.

So far we have described several determinants of detection apprehension: the personality of the liar and, before that, the reputation and character of the lie catcher. Equally important are the *stakes*—the perceived consequences for successful and unsuccessful attempts at deception. Although there is no direct empirical evidence for this assertion, research on the role of appraisal in the experience of emotion is consistent with our thinking (Lazarus, 1984). There is a simple rule: the greater the stakes, the more the detection apprehension. Applying this simple rule can be complicated because it is not always so easy to figure out what is at stake; for example, to some people winning is everything, so the stakes are always high. It is reasonable to presume that what is at stake in any deception situation may be so idiosyncratic that no outside observer would readily know.

Detection apprehension should be greater when the stakes involve avoiding punishment, not just earning a reward. When the decision to deceive is first made, the stakes usually involve obtaining rewards. The liar thinks primarily about what might be gained. An embezzler may think only about the monetary gain when he or she first chooses to lie. Once deceit has been underway for some time the rewards may no longer be available. The company may become aware of its losses and suspicious enough that the embezzler is prevented from taking more. At this point, the deceit might be maintained in order to avoid being caught, and avoiding punishment becomes the only stake. On the other hand, avoiding punishment may be the motive from the outset, if the target is suspicious or the liar has little confidence.

There are two kinds of punishment which are at stake in deceit: the punishment that lies in store if the lie fails; and the punishment for the very act of engaging in deception. Detection apprehension should be greater if both kinds of punishment are at stake. Sometimes the punishment for being caught deceiving can even be far worse than the punishment the lie was designed to avoid.

Even if the transgressor knows that the damage done if caught lying will be greater than the loss from admitting the transgression, the lie may be very tempting. Telling the truth brings immediate and certain losses, while telling a lie promises the possibility of avoiding all losses. The prospect of being spared immediate punishment may be so attractive that the liar may underestimate the likelihood that he or she will be caught in the lie. Recognition that confession would have been a better policy comes too late, when the lie has been maintained so long and with such elaboration that confession may no longer win a lesser punishment.

Sometimes there is little ambiguity about the relative costs of confession versus continued concealment. There are actions which are themselves so bad that confessing them wins little approval for having come forward, and concealing them adds little to the punishment which awaits the offender. Such is the case if the lie conceals child abuse, incest, murder, treason, or terrorism. Unlike the rewards possible for some repentant philanderers, forgiveness is not to be expected by those who confess these heinous crimes—although confession with contrition may lessen the punishment.

A final factor to consider about how the stakes influence detection apprehension is what is gained or lost by the target, not just by the liar. Usually the liar's gains are at the expense of the target. The embezzler gains what the employer loses. Stakes are not always equal; moreover, the stakes for the liar and the target can differ not just in amount but in kind. A philanderer may gain a little adventure, while the cuckolded spouse may lose tremendous self-respect. When the stakes differ for the liar and target, the stakes for either may determine the liar's detection apprehension. It depends upon whether the liar recognizes the difference and how it is evaluated.

Deception Guilt

Deception guilt refers to a feeling about lying, not the legal issue of whether someone is guilty or innocent. Deception guilt must also be distinguished from feelings of guilt about the content of a lie. Thus, a child may feel excitement about stealing the loose change off his parents' dresser, but feel guilt over lying to his or her parents to conceal the theft. This situation can be reversed as well—no guilt about lying to the parents, but guilt about stealing the money. Of course, some people feel guilt about both the act and the lie, and some people will not feel guilt about either. What is important is that it is not necessary to feel guilty about the content of a lie in order to feel guilty about lying.

Like the fear of being caught, deception guilt can vary in strength. It may be very mild, or so strong that the lie will fail because the deception guilt produces leakage or deception clues (Ekman & Friesen, 1969). When it becomes extreme, deception guilt is a torturing experience, undermining the sufferer's most fundamental feelings of self-worth. Relief from such severe deception guilt may motivate a confession despite the likelihood of punishment for misdeeds admitted. In fact the punishment may be sought by the person who confesses in order to alleviate the tortured feelings of guilt.

When the decision to lie is first made, people do not always accurately anticipate how much they may later suffer from deception guilt. Liars may not realize the impact of being thanked by their victims for their seeming helpfulness, or how they will feel when they see someone else blamed for their misdeeds—as in the recent case of the "gentleman bandit" who felt so guilty about someone else being prosecuted for his robberies that he turned himself in to the police. Another reason why liars underestimate how much deception guilt they will feel is that it is only with the passage of time that a liar may learn that one lie will not suffice, that the lie has to be repeated again and again, often with expanding fabrications in order to protect the original deceit (Mullaney, 1979).

Shame is closely related to guilt (Tomkins, 1963), but there is a key qualitative difference. No audience is needed for feelings of guilt, no one else need know for the guilty person is his own judge. Not so for shame. The humiliation of shame requires disapproval or ridicule by others (Campos & Barrett, 1984). If no one ever learns of a misdeed there will be no shame, but there still might be guilt. Of course there may be both. The distinction between shame and guilt is very important because these two emotions may tear a person in opposite directions. The wish to relieve guilt may motivate a confession, but the wish to avoid the humiliation of shame may prevent it.

There exists a group of individuals who fail to feel any guilt or shame about their misdeeds; these people have been referred to as sociopaths or psychopaths (Hare, 1970). For these individuals, the lack of guilt or shame pervades all or most aspects of their lives. Experts disagree about whether the lack of guilt and shame is due to upbringing or some biological determinants (MacMillan & Kofoed, 1984; Schmauk, 1970; Vaillant, 1975). There is agreement that the psychopath's lack of guilt about lying and lack of fear of being caught will make it more difficult for a target to detect a psychopath's lies.

Conversely, some people are especially vulnerable to shame about lying and deception guilt; for example, people who have been very strictly brought up to believe lying is one of the most terrible sins. Those with less strict upbringing, that did not particularly condemn lying, could more generally have been instilled with strong, pervasive guilt feelings. Such guilty people appear to seek experiences in which they can intensify their guilt, and stand shamefully exposed to others; this appears to be the case for psychiatric patients suffering from generalized anxiety disorders. Unfortunately, unlike the psychopathic personality, there has been very little research about guilt-prone individuals.

Whenever the deceiver does not share social values with the victim, odds are there will not be much deception guilt. People feel less guilty about lying to those they think are wrongdoers. A philanderer whose marital partner is cold and unwilling in bed might not feel guilty in lying about an affair. A similar principle is at work to explain why a diplomat or spy does not feel guilty about misleading the other side. In all these situations, the liar and the target do not share common goals or values.

Lying is authorized in most of these examples—each of these individuals appeals to a well-defined social norm which legitimizes deceiving an opponent. There is little guilt about such authorized deceits when the targets are from opposing sides, and hold different values. There also may be authorization to deceive targets who are not opponents, who share values with the deceiver. Physicians may not feel guilty about deceiving their patients if they think it is for the patient's own good. Giving a patient a placebo, a sugar pill identified as a useful drug, is an old, time-honored, medical deceit. If the patient feels better, or at least stops hassling the doctor for an unneeded drug which might actually be harmful, many physicians believe that the lie is justified. In this case, the patient benefits from the lie, and not the doctor. If a liar thinks he is not gaining from the lie he probably will not feel any deception guilt.

Even selfish deceits may not produce deception guilt when the lie is authorized. Poker players do not feel deception guilt about bluffing (but they do feel detection apprehension; Frank, 1989). The same is true about bargaining whether in a Middle East bazaar, Wall Street, or in the local real estate agent's office. The home owner who asks more for his house than he will actually sell it for will not feel guilty if he gets his asking price. This lie is authorized. Because the participants expect misinformation, and not the truth, bargaining and poker are not necessarily lies (Ekman, 1985). These situations by their nature provide prior notification that no one will be entirely truthful.

Deception guilt is most likely when lying is not authorized. Deception guilt should be most severe when the target is trusting, not expecting to be misled because honesty is expected between liar and target. In such opportunistic deceits, guilt about lying will be greater if the target suffers at least as much as the liar gains. Even then there will not be much, if any, deception guilt unless there are at least some shared values between target and liar. A student turning in a late assignment may not feel guilty about lying to the professor if the student feels the professor sets unreachable standards and assigns undoable workloads. This student may feel fear of being caught in a lie, but he or she may not feel deception guilt. Even though the student disagrees with the professor about the workload and other matters, if the student still cares about the professor he or she may feel shame if the lie is discovered. Shame requires some respect for those who disapprove; otherwise disapproval brings forth anger or contempt, not shame.

Liars feel less guilty when their targets are impersonal or totally anonymous. A customer who conceals from the check-out clerk that he or she was undercharged for an expensive item will feel less guilty if he or she does not know the clerk. If the clerk is the owner, or if it is a small family owned store, the lying customer will feel more guilty than he or she will if it is one of a large chain of supermarkets. It is easier to indulge the guilt-reducing fantasy that the target is not really hurt, does not really care, will not even notice the lie, or even deserves or wants to be misled, if the target is anonymous (Wolk & Henley, 1970).

Often there will be an inverse relationship between deception guilt and detection apprehension. What lessens guilt about the lie increases fear of being caught. When deceits are authorized there should be less deception guilt, yet the authorization usually increases the stakes, thus making detection apprehension high. In a high stakes poker game there is high detection apprehension and low deception guilt (Frank, 1989). The employer who lies to his employee whom he has come to suspect of embezzling, concealing his suspicions to catch him in the crime, also is likely to feel high detection apprehension but low deception guilt.

While there are exceptions, most people find the experience of guilt so toxic that they seek ways to diminish it. There are many ways to justify deceit. It can be considered retaliation for injustice. A nasty or mean target can be said not to deserve honesty. "The boss was so stingy, he didn't reward me for all the work I did, so I took some myself." Or the liar can blame the victim of his or her lies; for example, Machiavellian personality types tend to see their victims as so gullible that they bring lies upon themselves (Christie & Geis, 1970).

Two other justifications for lying which reduce deception guilt were mentioned earlier. A noble purpose or job requirement is one—as in the case of the diplomat or the spy. The other justification is to protect the target—as in the case of the doctor. Sometimes the liar may go so far as to claim that the target was willing. If the target cooperated in the deceit, knew the truth all along but pretended not to, then in a sense there was no lie, and the liar is free of any deception guilt. A willing target helps the deceiver maintain the deceit, overlooking any behavioral betrayals of the lie. People often cooperate in being misled, as in polite social encounters (Rosenthal & DePaulo, 1979). For example, politeness requires a hostess to accept without scrutiny a guest's excuse for an early departure.

An unwilling target may after a time become a willing one in order to avoid the costs of discovering deceit. Imagine the plight of the government official who begins to suspect that the lover to whom he has been trusting information about his work might be a spy. A job recruiter may similarly become the willing victim of a fraudulent job applicant, once the applicant is hired, rather than acknowledge his own mistaken judgment.

Duping Delight

The fear of being caught in a lie and the guilt aroused by lying are negative feelings. Lying can also produce positive feelings. The lie may be viewed as a proud accomplishment. The liar may feel excitement, either when anticipating the challenge or during the very moment of lying, when success is not yet certain. Afterward there may be the pleasure that comes with relief, pride in the achievement, or feelings of smug contempt toward the target. Duping delight refers to any or all of these feelings which can, if not concealed, betray the deceit.

An innocent example of duping delight occurs when kidding takes the form of misleading a gullible friend. The kidder has to conceal his duping delight even though his performance may in large part be directed to others who are appreciating how well the gullible person is being duped.

Like all emotions, duping delight can vary in strength. It may be totally absent, almost insignificant compared to the amount of detection apprehension which is felt, or duping delight may be so great that some behavioral sign of it leaks. People may confess their deception in order to share their delight in having put one over. Criminals have been known to reveal their crime to friends, strangers, even to the police, in order to be acknowledged and appreciated as having been clever enough to pull off a particular deceit. Virtually every James Bond film features a scene where the villain, after capturing Bond, cannot resist divulging his entire diabolical plan to Bond before he has Bond put to death.

There are several factors that may enhance duping delight. If the person being deceived has the reputation of being difficult to fool, then this increased challenge adds to the liar's delight in duping this person. The presence of others who know what is going on can also increase the likelihood of duping delight. When the audience is present, enjoying the liar's performance, the liar may have the most duping delight and the hardest time suppressing any sign of it. When one child lies to another while others watch, the liar may so enjoy observing how he is entertaining his buddies that his delight bursts forth ending the whole matter.

Some people may be much more prone to duping delight. No scientist has yet studied such people or even verified that they do exist. Yet it seems obvious that, like James Bond villains, some people boast more than others, and that braggarts might be more vulnerable than others to duping delight.

While lying, a person may feel duping delight, deception guilt, and detection apprehension—all at once or in succession. Consider poker again. In a bluff, when a player has poor cards but is pretending to have such good cards that the others will fold, there may be detection apprehension if the pot has gotten very high. As the bluffer watches each player cave in, he may also feel duping delight. Since misinformation is authorized there should be no deception guilt as long as the poker player does not cheat. Yet an embezzler might feel all three emotions: delight in how he or she has fooled fellow employees and employer; apprehension at moments when he or she thinks there might be some suspicion; and, perhaps, guilt about having broken the law and violated trust shown in him or her by the company.

CAVEATS

We maintain that there are no behavioral clues that are specific to lying. There are two recurrent errors that a lie detector can make when deciding upon the honesty of a potential liar; these have been called by Ekman (1985) the *Othello error* and the *idiosyncrasy error*.

The first error that a lie detector can make is the *Othello error*. Like Shakespeare's tragic hero—who misinterprets his wife's fear and distress over the possibility that Othello may kill her, as a sign that she is lying to him—the lie detector disbelieves the truth and fails to consider the stress that his or her disbelief puts upon the truthful person. For example, the truthful person's fear of being disbelieved may be misinterpreted by the lie detector as a fear of being caught. Moreover, some people have such strong unresolved guilt about other matters that these feelings may be aroused whenever they are accused of any wrongdoing, and these signs of guilt may be misinterpreted as signs of deception guilt.

It may also be the case that truthful people will feel scorn toward those they know are falsely accusing them, or excitement about the challenge of proving their accusers wrong, or pleasure in anticipating their vindication. These feelings may produce signs that resemble signs of duping delight. Although the reasons would differ, either the liar or the truthful person might feel surprised, angry, disappointed, distressed, or disgusted by the lie detector's suspicions or questions.

The second error—the *idiosyncrasy error* (originally called the "Brokaw Hazard" by Ekman, 1985)—involves the failure of the lie detector to take account of individual differences in a potential liar's behavior. This type of error may cause the lie detector to both disbelieve the truth as well as falsely believe a lie. For example, many lie detectors believe that a liar cannot make eye contact while telling a lie, even though deception research has shown that eye contact is not related to deception (DePaulo, Stone, & Lassiter, 1985). Thus, a person who never makes eye contact when he or she speaks will appear deceptive to a lie detector when in fact this is the person's normal interpersonal style. Many of the thinking clues to deceit mentioned earlier fall into this same category; that is, many people normally speak in a circumlocutory fashion, make speech errors, or make either long or short pauses in speech. There are substantial differences among all individuals in all of these behaviors, and these differences may produce mistakes in both disbelieving the truth and believing a lie.

A partial solution to this problem is for the lie detector to base his or her decisions on the observed *changes* in a suspected liar's behavior. The lie detector must compare the person's usual behavior to his or her behavior when under suspicion. This is why a person is more likely to be mislead in a first meeting with a deceiver as compared to ensuing meetings because in the first meeting there is no basis for comparing changes in a suspected deceiver's behavior (see Brandt, Miller, & Hocking, 1980; Frank, 1989; O'Sullivan, Ekman, & Friesen, 1988). However, it is not always the case that detecting deception is easier from those with whom we have more contact; spouses, good friends, and family members may develop blind spots or preconceptions that interfere with accurate perceptions of the behavioral clues to deceit.

Analyzing which emotions a particular deceiver is likely to feel and which emotions a truthful person might feel about being suspected or disbelieved can help to identify a liar. Such an analysis may isolate unambiguous signs of honesty or deceit and may alert the lie detector to the behaviors that must be discovered.

SUMMARY

Guilt, fear, and delight all can be shown in facial expression, the voice, or body movement, even when the liar is trying to conceal them. There are certainly specific and reliable signs of these emotions in the facial expressions and voices of these deceivers (e.g., Ekman & Friesen, 1974; Ekman, O'Sullivan, Friesen, & Scherer, 1991; Frank, Ekman, & Friesen, 1991). Even if there is no nonverbal leakage, the struggle to prevent it may also produce a deception clue.

Thus, a lie detector must be aware of the circumstances that may elevate or deflate the three factors which make a lie detectable, regardless of whether the liar shows thinking clues, is lying about feelings, or is having feelings about lying. Below is a summary listing of the situations in which evidence for the behavioral clues to deceit will be strongest.

The evidence of *thinking clues* will be greatest when:

- The liar does not anticipate when he or she will have to lie.
- The liar is not very clever or inventive.
- The liar should know the answer to the posed questions.

The evidence of *lying about feelings* will be greatest when:

- The lie involves emotions felt at the moment.
- The truly felt emotion is strong.
- The liar fails to show reliable clues to the emotion he or she is feigning.

Fear of being caught will be greatest when:

- The target has a reputation for being tough to fool.
- The target starts out being suspicious.
- The liar has had little practice and no record of success.
- The liar is especially vulnerable to the fear of being caught.
- The stakes are high.
- Both rewards and punishments are at stake; or, if it is only one or the other, then it is punishment which is at stake.
- The punishment for being caught lying is great, or the punishment for what the lie is about is so great that there is no incentive to confess.

- The target in no way benefits from the lie.

Deception guilt will be greatest when:

- The target is unwilling.
- The deceit is totally selfish, and the target derives no benefit from being misled and loses as much or more than the liar gains.
- The deceit is unauthorized, and the situation is one in which honesty is authorized.
- The liar has not been practicing the deceit for a long time.
- The liar and target share social values.
- The liar is personally acquainted with the target.
- The target cannot easily be faulted as mean or gullible.
- There is no reason for the target to expect to be misled; just the opposite, the liar has acted to win confidence in his trustworthiness.

Finally, *duping delight* will be greatest when:

- The target poses a challenge having a reputation for being difficult to fool.
- The lie is a challenge, because of either what must be concealed or the nature of what must be fabricated.
- Others are watching or know about the lie and appreciate the liar's skillful performance.

It needs to be reiterated that these behavioral clues which betray a lie are not specific to lying, and thus the lie detector must beware of making either the Othello error or the idiosyncrasy error. The simplest suggestion is for the lie detector to try to understand what reasons might the possible liar have for showing these signs of emotion besides lying. Ultimately, it is our hope that people who interpret potential clues to deceit or truthfulness would do so with great care because not only do lies fail, but people fail to lie.

Acknowledgments

The research presented in this chapter was supported by a Research Scientist Award # MH06092 to the first author. The second author is supported by a NIMH National Research Service Award # MH09827.

References

Brandt, D. R., Miller, G. R., & Hocking, J. E. (1980). The truth–deception attribution: Effects of familiarity on the ability of observers to detect deception. *Human Communication Research, 6,* 99–110.

Campos, J. J., & Barrett, K. C. (1984). Toward a new understanding of emotions and their development. In C. E. Izard, J. Kagan, & R. B. Zajonc (Eds.), *Emotions, cognition and behavior* (pp. 229–263). London: Cambridge University Press.

Christie, R., & Geis, F. L. (1970). *Studies in Machiavellianism.* New York: Academic Press.

Davidson, R. J., Ekman, P., Saron, C., Senulius, J., & Friesen, W. V. (1991). Approach-withdrawal and cerebral asymmetry: Emotional expression and brain physiology I. *Journal of Personality and Social Psychology, 58,* 330–341.

DePaulo, B. M., Lanier, K., & Davis, T. (1983). Detecting deceit of the motivated liar. *Journal of Personality and Social Psychology, 45,* 1096–1103.

DePaulo, B. M., Stone, J. I., & Lassiter, D. (1985). Deceiving and detecting deceit. In B. R. Schlenker (Ed.), *The self and social life* (pp. 323–370). New York: McGraw-Hill.

Ekman, P. (1985). *Telling lies.* New York: W. W. Norton.

Ekman, P., Davidson, R. J., & Friesen, W. V. (1991). The Duchenne smile: Emotional expression and brain physiology II. *Journal of Personality and Social Psychology, 58,* 342–353.

Ekman, P., & Friesen, W. V. (1969). Nonverbal leakage and clues to deception. *Psychiatry, 32,* 88–105.

Ekman, P., & Friesen, W. V. (1974). Detecting deception from the body or face. *Journal of Personality and Social Psychology, 29,* 288–298.

Ekman, P., & Friesen, W. V. (1975). *Unmasking the face.* Englewood Cliffs, NJ: Prentice-Hall.

Ekman, P., Friesen, W. V., & O'Sullivan, M. (1988). Smiles when lying. *Journal of Personality and Social Psychology, 54,* 414–420.

Ekman, P., Friesen, W. V., & Scherer, K. (1976). Body movement and voice pitch in deceptive interaction. *Semiotica, 16,* 23–27.

Ekman, P., O'Sullivan, M., Friesen, W. V., & Scherer, K. (1991). Face, voice, and body in detecting deceit. *Journal of Nonverbal Behavior, 15,* 125–135.

Frank, M. G. (1989). *Human lie detection ability as a function of the liar's motivation.* Unpublished doctoral dissertation, Cornell University.

Frank, M. G., Ekman, P., & Friesen, W. V. (in press). Behavioral markers and recognizability of the smile of enjoyment. *Journal of Personality and Social Psychology.*

Fridja, N. H. (1986). *The emotions.* Cambridge, UK: Cambridge University Press.

Hager, J. C., & Ekman, P. (1985). The asymmetry of facial action is inconsistent with models of hemispheric specialization. *Psychophysiology*, 22, 307–318.

Hare, R. D. (1970). *Psychopathy: Theory and research*. New York: Wiley.

Hood, W. (1982). *Mole*. New York: W. W. Norton.

Lazarus, R. S. (1984). On the primacy of cognition. *American Psychologist*, 39, 124–129.

MacMillan, J., & Kofoed, L. (1984). Sociobiology and antisocial personality: An alternative perspective. *Journal of Mental Disease*, 172, 701–706.

Mullaney, R. (1979). *The third way—the interroview*. Unpublished manuscript.

O'Sullivan, M., Ekman, P., & Friesen, W. V. (1988). The effect of behavioral comparison in detecting deception. *Journal of Nonverbal Behavior*, 12, 203–215.

Rosenthal, R., & DePaulo, B. M. (1979). Sex differences in accommodation in nonverbal communication. In R. Rosenthal (Ed.), *Skill in nonverbal communication: Individual differences* (pp. 68–103). Cambridge, MA: Oelgeschlager.

Schmauk, F. J. (1970). Punishment, arousal, and avoidance learning in sociopaths. *Journal of Abnormal Psychology*, 76, 325–335.

Swann, W. B., Griffin, J. J., Predmore, S. C., & Gaines, B. (1987). Cognitive-affective crossfire: When self-consistency meets self-enhancement. *Journal of Personality and Social Psychology*, 52, 881–889.

Tomkins, S. S. (1963). *Affect, imagery, and consciousness: The negative affects* (Vol. 2). New York: Springer Publishing Co.

Vaillant, G. E. (1975). Sociopathy as a human process: A viewpoint. *Archives of General Psychiatry*, 32, 178–183.

Wolk, R. L., & Henley, A. (1970). *The right to lie*. New York: Peter Wyden.

Zuckerman, M., & Driver, R. E. (1985). Telling lies: Verbal and nonverbal correlates of deception. In A. W. Siegman & S. Feldstein (Eds.), *Multichannel integration of nonverbal behavior* (pp. 129–147). Hillsdale, NJ: Erlbaum.

10
Understanding Malingering:
Motivation, Method, and Detection

P. RANDALL KROPP
RICHARD ROGERS

Malingering is defined as a deliberate attempt to feign a disability or illness in order to achieve some secondary gain or reward. The malingerer is typically viewed by the public as someone attempting to get away with something—to "dupe" the system. This generally negative image is generated both by the connotation of the word itself, with its Latin root "mal" (i.e., evil), and by mass media reports of high profile cases: the murderer trying to plead insanity, or the healthy worker trying to defraud an insurance company. While it can be argued that this unflattering view is deserved in some cases, it may very well be overly simplistic in others. The primary goal of this chapter is to provide an overview of malingering to facilitate a better understanding of this complex condition.

Unlike other forms of lying described in this book, malingering, in its more blatant forms, is rarely seen in the general public. Certain exceptions to this observation do occur (see Table 1) and some are even considered socially acceptable. For example, many individuals invoke the excuse of feigned fatigue or illness when turning down sexual overtures and social commitments.

We will devote most of our attention to blatant forms of malingering for two reasons. First, nearly all the available literature addresses these severe cases. Second, subtle forms of malingering are very difficult to reliably define. Most of us experience some degree of discomfort much of the time. Who is competent to specify when a purported ache, muscle tension, or pain is sufficiently spurious to be classified as malingering? Nevertheless, we will speculate about everyday life situations throughout the chapter to help illustrate the phenomenon of malingering.

The chapter includes a description of some common "types" of malingering and discusses models of what motivates the malingerer. It

201

Table 1. Everyday Examples of Malingering

Feigned deficit	Possible Motivation
Illness or fatigue "stopped" employee from meeting a deadline.	Avoid disapproval or censure.
Pain, illness, or fatigue "prevented" sexual relations.	Avoid potential conflict over disinterest in sex.
Anxiety, tension or nerves "impaired" student's performance on a test.	Obtain a special consideration such as a make-up exam.
Illness or fatigue "forced" a cancellation of a social obligation.	Provide an opportunity for more enjoyable activity.

also includes a discussion of personality variables associated with malingering, with particular attention to psychopathic personality. It then focuses on strategies used by malingerers and concludes with a review of methods used by clinicians to detect feigned mental illness. Although the focus is primarily on the malingering of mental illness, the feigning of physical disability will also be included where applicable. Our aim is to explore the malingering phenomenon from the perspectives of both the "patient" and the clinician.

WHAT IS MALINGERING?

As mentioned, the distinguishing feature of the malingerer is that he/she is exaggerating or fabricating symptoms in order to achieve some external goal. The nature of the "rewards" for successful malingering varies across individuals and settings, but certain examples have received considerable public scrutiny. In clinical settings, for example, there is often motivation on behalf of the patient to exaggerate symptomatology in order to receive injury compensation. Insurance agencies and compensation boards typically invest substantial effort and expense to expose these individuals. Failure to do so can result in the unnecessary depletion of health and disability insurance resources. Malingering in such situations has sometimes been referred to as *compensation neurosis* (Weighill, 1983). This label typically describes cases in which physical or psychological disability persists long after expected recovery from injury. Symptoms in this condition generally exceed the physical findings resulting from medical examination and other investigative procedures.

Mental health issues arising in the legal system is another context commonly associated with feigned illness. Here the potential gain can be even more far reaching for the malingerer. For example, being found "unfit" to stand trial can serve to delay the trial date, increase media coverage, and possibly render the key witnesses unavailable (Roesch & Golding, 1980). Moreover, a verdict of not guilty by reason of insanity can result in an individual avoiding a prison sentence or, in exceptional cases, the death penalty. In fact, the role of malingering in the criminal context is extremely controversial. A number of surveys conducted throughout the United States indicate that the majority of the public believes the insanity defense is an often used strategy for getting away with a crime. The outcry following the acquittal of John Hinckley for the attempted murder of then president Ronald Reagan is illustrative of public suspiciousness. It should be noted, however, that the insanity defense is seldom used, and even when it is attempted, it is rarely successful.

A well known example of a case of malingering in a legal context occurred in the homicide trial of Kenneth Bianchi, better known as the "Hillside Strangler." Mr. Bianchi was charged with and ultimately convicted of a series of stranglings in Washington State. During the pretrial process, he claimed amnesia for the periods surrounding the crimes. In addition, he claimed to have a multiple personalities, and succeeded in convincing several experts that he had this rare condition. It was eventually proved that Bianchi was simulating these symptoms and had been planning his defense for years.

Factitious Disorders

Malingering is closely related to a group of conditions referred to in the medical literature as the *factitious disorders* (Rogers, Bagby, & Rector, 1989). The word factitious is defined as artificial or unnatural. Factitious disorders are therefore characterized by false physical and/or psychological complaints that are under voluntary control. What distinguishes these disorders from malingering itself are the motives of the patient. In the case of factitious disorders, the goal of the individual is to maintain the role of the patient; that is, there is no recognizable benefit from the symptom fabrication other than the attention received from health care professionals and facilities. The distinction between malingering and factitious disorder underscores a less hostile attitude taken toward individuals who feign illness solely to gain attention from the medical profession. In fact, their sustained motivation to be a patient results, albeit reluctantly, in the diagnosis of factitious disorder and the tenuous achievement of patient status.

A well-publicized example of these disorders is the chronic presentation of *Munchausen's syndrome*. Patients with Munchausen's have a long history of physical complaints that cannot be confirmed by medical assessment. Such patients are typically admitted to the hospital with a dramatic and marginally believable account of symptoms such as severe stomach problems, chronic pain, or neurological illness. In cases where the patient desires surgical intervention, there often exist multiple scars from previous surgeries. In extreme cases of gastrointestinal complaints, Munchausen patients have occasionally been referred to as having "gridiron" abdomens as a colorful description of scar tissue resulting from multiple exploratory operations. Another complicating feature of Munchausen's syndrome can be the patient's dependence on pharmaceutical intervention (e.g., pain medication).

A disturbing variation of this disorder is *Munchausen syndrome by proxy*. This term has been used to describe a condition in which caretakers, typically parents, repeatedly give false accounts of the health of their children to medical professionals. According to Meadow (1977) the state of affairs may reach the extreme situation whereby the parent will induce the symptoms in the child. For example, the parent may attempt to worsen the child's condition by producing seizures, neglecting true illness, or by administering toxic substances. As in Munchausen's syndrome, the parent/caretaker may feel that the production of symptoms in the child is the only means available to maintain contact with the health care system. Munchausen's by proxy achieves the "goal" of satisfying the dependency needs of the caretaker.

WHY DO PEOPLE MALINGER?

Early writers proposed a psychopathogenic process of malingering in which dissimulation represented an ineffectual coping with an underlying disorder. This *pathogenic model* originated with Carl Jung in 1903, was elaborated upon by Sigmund Freud, and continues to have its modern day adherents. According to this model, malingering is seen as the early stages of a more serious disease. This view has been widely criticized, however, as it became increasingly apparent that many malingerers did not subsequently become mentally ill. Contrary to expectations, some showed remarkable improvement in their problems once an external goal was achieved.

With the loss in popularity of the pathogenic explanations, the medical and psychological literature has seen the emergence of a *criminogenic model* of malingering (Rogers, 1990). Thus, there has been a shift from a generally sympathetic view of the malingerer as an unwitting "victim" of his/her disorder, to a more punitive perception of the malingerer as a deliberate "con." The criminogenic model forms the basis of our current classification system of mental disorders. More specifically, the American Psychiatric Association (1987, p. 360) proposed that any combination of the following factors raises a high index of suspicion for malingering:

1. Medicolegal context of presentation, for example, the person's being referred by his or her attorney to the physician for examination.
2. Marked discrepancy between the person's claimed distress or disability and the objective findings.
3. Lack of cooperation with diagnostic evaluation and in complying with prescribed treatment regimen.
4. The presence of antisocial personality disorder (APD).

This model provides a combination of characterological variables (antisocial personality disorder), contextual variables (medicolegal evaluations), and interpersonal variables (uncooperativeness). The unifying theme of these factors is that of "badness," namely, a bad person, in a bad situation, who is a bad participant. The APA offered no explanation for this paradigmatic shift and by adopting such a model contributes, at least implicitly, to the prevailing negative public image of the malingerer. Available research would suggest that only a minority of malingerers have one or more of these indices (Rogers, 1990) and that the adoption of this model is, at best, premature. Moreover, no literature exists that links antisocial personality disorders with malingering (this will be discussed at length in the next section). In addition, the use of uncooperativeness as a factor in establishing malingering is illogical given the substantial percentage of patients who are either unable or unwilling to participate actively in their assessment and/or treatment. It is simply an overinclusive criterion, and like APD, lacks an established empirical support.

We believe that a reconceptualization of malingering is necessary with a return to a less pejorative view. From the perspective of the would-be malingerer, feigning an illness may be an adaptive effort to deal with difficult circumstances. Rogers (1990) described this explanation as an *adaptational model*. Assumptions of this adaptational model are threefold: (1) a person perceives the evaluation/treatment as involuntary or adversarial; (2) the person perceives that he/she has either something to lose from self-disclosure or something to gain from malingering; and (3) the person does not perceive a more effective means to achieve his/her desired goal.

Malingering in the armed forces offers an instructive example of the adaptational model. Concern for feigned mental illness increases dramatically during wartime. In such times, an adversarial situation (such as a military draft) creates potential rewards for "dodging," namely, avoiding combat and possible death. For example, it has been noted that in World War I the Austrian army experienced only a handful of malingerers in the early stages of the war, but that a mass phenomenon, estimated at 100,000, occurred as the casualties mounted. Similarly, it has been observed that in criminal forensic settings, particularly when defendants are faced with very serious charges, many more individuals feign mental illness than under comparatively benign circumstances. Finally, it can be speculated that many inner city hospital admissions are related to somewhat desperate attempts by homeless individuals to obtain a decent meal, accommodations, and a respite from extremely difficult living conditions.

This model avoids the pejorative and moralistic assumptions about the malingerer, placing less "blame" on the person, and advocates a contextual understanding of the malingering process. Such a model recognizes the complexity of individual circumstances and focuses on the adversarial nature of these circumstances. Seen in this light, malingering may be construed as one of many possible options for the individual who finds him/herself in a very difficult situation.

The adaptational model is also appropriate for explaining the examples of "everyday life" malingering given in Table 1. As a way of placing this point in perspective, it is suggested that the reader think of instances where he/she was tempted to feign illness. Many will recall phoning into work sick and being less than truthful about the severity of symptoms. Indeed, the well-known excuse, "not tonight I have a headache," is another all too familiar example of malingering in everyday life. These cases can all be construed as arising out of difficult situations for which malingering is the most desirable solution. For example, feigning a headache to avoid sexual relations may allow the malingerer to (1) avoid an unenjoyable sexual encounter, (2) postpone inevitable discussion about a conflict in the relationship, or (3) avoid the potential argument resulting from being assertive.

WHO MALINGERS?

The above discussion suggests that everyone malingers, or at least exaggerates illness, occasionally. Some research has begun to address whether some individuals are more prone to malingering than others. This research has only focused on more severe cases of malingering due to the serious consequences described earlier. The question is: Who should we suspect? Certainly the contextual factors discussed (legal cases, insurance claims) offer some clues. But they are not enough. Why, for example, does not everyone before the court or applying for worker's compensation pretend to be more physically or mentally ill? It may be that, given the adversarial context described above, certain individuals may be more inclined to choose malingering as an option. Indeed, the clinical puzzle of malingerers and the difficulties in their detection have led many researchers and clinicians to hypothesize personality variables, or aspects of the person, which might be related to successful malingering. Unfortunately, not much is known about the characteristics of the typical malingerer; further research is necessary.

An example of a possible direction in this area has been alluded to above. Much suggestion has been made that a certain type of condition—antisocial personality disorder or APD—may be related to the tendency and ability to malinger. As noted, the DSM-III-R lists this as one of the conditions under which to suspect malingering. Despite the formulations implicating these individuals, however, we have also noted the lack of empirical evidence supporting this link.

One of the reasons for a failure to establish a link may be that the diagnosis of APD is overinclusive. For example, because the disorder is based primarily on the presence of antisocial behavior, this is an extremely common diagnosis. Prevalence estimates of APD have reached as high as 75% in many prison/forensic settings, making it impossible to use it as a predictor of feigned illness (i.e., it is impractical to suspect 75% of a population, especially in the light of the low base rate of feigned illness). There may, however, be reason to believe that a subgroup of the antisocial group, namely, the psychopathic personalities, may be more prone to malinger.

The term "psychopath" is an often-used term in the media and entertainment industries. However, it is a poorly understood term. Typically, the psychopath is portrayed as psychotic, violent and unpredictable—usually randomly preying on his/her victims. The consensus in mental health circles is considerably different. The psychopathic (or sociopathic) personality is generally described as an individual who has little empathy for others and uses them to his/her advantage. Often they are superficially charming, manipulative, and deceitful. The psychopath may or may not get in trouble with the law, but if antisocial behavior occurs, there is typically no remorse. Interestingly, the Hillside Strangler, described earlier, closely fits this description. However, many other noncriminals—perhaps successful businesspersons, lawyers, etc.—have certain psychopathic tendencies. We have included this description because there are a number of intuitive reasons to suspect a relationship between psychopathy and malingering.

First, a number of clinical and theoretical accounts suggest a connection between the two. Most clinical descriptions of the psychopath make reference to a tendency and ability to lie, deceive, and manipulate others (Cleckley, 1982). Explanations for deception in psychopaths range from sociobiological adaptation to cognitive and/or language dysfunction (Hare, Williamson, & Harpur, 1988). It follows from these assumed abilities/tendencies that the psychopath is a prime candidate to feign mental illness. It is noteworthy that such descriptions suggest the psychopath not only can malinger (e.g., manipulativeness), but also has a tendency to try (e.g., chronic lying).

A second reason to investigate a psychopathy–malingering link is that psychopathic features are highly represented in a number of criminal populations. For example, the estimates of the incidence of psychopathy in both penitentiary and forensic psychiatric populations have ranged from 15% to 30% (Hart & Hare, 1989). Thus, with the secondary gain associated with malingering in these populations, and from the perspective of an adaptational model, the psychopathic individual may have the motivation as well as the capacity to feign mental illness.

Despite these theoretical connections, research addressing the relationship between psychopathy and malingering has been scarce. For example, Sierles (1984) reported a significant correlation between scores on a malingering index and a very general measure of sociopathic behavior patterns. Similar findings were reported by Hare, Hart, and Forth (1989) who found small correlations between a measure of psychopathy (Psychopathy Checklist: Hare, 1991) and a tendency to claim obvious symptoms of psychopathology on the MMPI (for a description of the MMPI, see a later section on detection of malingering). Alternatively, Rogers, Gillis, and Bagby (1990) did not find a relationship between antisocial behavior and ability to malinger in a simulation design. However, this latter study used a fairly broad definition of antisocial behavior that did not necessarily discriminate among groups based on key sociopathic variables such as manipulativeness and lying. As noted, it is likely that stringent criteria for psychopathy is necessary to detect differences between psychopaths and others in malingering tendencies/abilities. Thus, taken together, the more rigorous diagnoses of psychopathic behavior in the first studies may offer tentative support for a psychopathy–malingering link.

We are currently conducting research, using stringent criteria for assessing psychopathy, that will help to unravel this puzzle. We hope the result will enable us to determine whether or not psychopathic individuals are more prone to dissimulation or more effective at malingering. The reader may wish to think about whether or not he/she knows anyone that fits the description of the psychopath (i.e., manipulative, superficial, lacking empathy, etc.) and consider if this person might be more prone to malingering. It might be the case, in other words, that noncriminal psychopathic individuals may be more prone to malinger in everyday life as well. These individuals' lack of concern for the consequences of their actions and lack of empathy may allow them to feign illness without the guilt or remorse that most people experience.

It should be emphasized that the investigation of a psychopathy–malingering link represents only one possible direction in the exploration of personality features of malingerers. It may be useful, for example, to explore whether or not malingering is related to hypochondriacal tendencies (i.e., individuals who deal with conflicts through physical complaints). Other possibilities would be to explore the relationship between malingering and pathological lying or Machiavellian traits. Finally, it might be that histrionic individuals—that is, those with an overdramatic flair and tendency to draw attention to themselves—may be more prone to exaggeration, if not malingering.

HOW DO PEOPLE MALINGER?: THE MALINGERER'S PERSPECTIVE

Despite the great importance of this question, very little is known about the ways in which the malingerer operates. Again this is likely to vary from individual to individual, in line with his/her own perception of mental illness and its corollary behaviors. This question is typically difficult to research since there are few identified malingers with whom to investigate strategies. Nonetheless, selected case studies provide a few answers. We know for example that Mr. Bianchi chose to educate himself extensively about the nature and presentation of multiple personality disorder. His feigning was obviously a well planned and sophisticated effort. We suspect, however, that most malingerers do not make such a substantial effort to plan their course of action. In fact, the majority of those feigning illness are probably quite naive.

Some suggestion of the naivete of attempted malingerers comes from research done by the current authors at the Clarke Institute of Psychiatry (Rogers et al., 1990; Kropp & Rogers, 1991). This research has focused on both criminal defendants and college students. We have conducted a number of studies in which we asked a number of individuals to pretend that they had a mental illness. The volunteers were given time to prepare and in some cases given material to read about various mental disorders. In all cases, the subjects of our research were considered psychologically knowledgeable, as they were either taking courses in psychology at university, or were incarcerated in a treatment facility for criminals with mental health problems.

After giving the research participants the instructions to malinger, we conducted interviews using a questionnaire designed by one of the authors (R. R.) to detect malingering. In all cases, a modest reward was offered as incentive for making a good effort at appearing mentally ill. Despite the presumed psychological sophistication of the volunteers, these individuals rarely came even close to giving a convincing presentation. Surprisingly, however, we have found in post-test interviews that the majority of "malingerers" (approximately 90%) believed they did a good job at fooling the examiner. We interpret this marked discrepancy as possibly representing an inaccurate and fairly simplistic public image of true mental illness.

These subjects were also asked a series of questions about how they attempted to fool the interviewer. Both college students and inmates commonly pretended to be psychotic in some way. They would try to present that they were paranoid and experiencing hallucinations. Other commonly feigned problems were anxiety and depression. Again, however, our subjects generally described very unsophisticated strategies. Some of the more common strategies included: (1) answering all questions in the opposite direction to the truth, (2) offering ridiculous answers to straightforward questions, (3) constantly playing with a pen, pencil, or paper, (4) trying to talk as little as possible, (5) ignoring certain questions, and (6) contradicting themselves often.

We refer to these strategies as "unsophisticated" because they generally result in presentations very different from those of truly mentally ill individuals. The literature indicates, for example, that such behaviors are relatively infrequent in bona fide patients. These observations must be tempered by the admission that the incentive for the volunteers to malinger was relatively low in our research when compared to the far-reaching consequences for real-life malingerers. We suspect that more effort would be made to learn about the feigned illness if large sums of money or an insanity plea were at stake. Nonetheless, it is significant that these individuals rarely could "fool" the interview, despite having considerable experience with mental health issues.

As mentioned, our research participants had a generally overinflated view of their ability to feign mental illness. Many of the volunteers felt that it was "easy" to do. The results of this and other research suggest the contrary. The lack of success in simulation studies is likely partly due to the fact that malingering is difficult to do. It takes careful planning, and the patience and perseverance to maintain a convincing presentation over a long period of time. Interestingly, many of the inmates contacted for research purposes have commented that they have considered malingering at times in their lives, but have been deterred because of the sheer annoyance of constantly having to pretend they were someone that they were not. The process is laborious, anxiety-provoking and, in many cases in the criminal justice system, not even to the malingerer's advantage. For example, it may simply result in being incarcerated in an equally restrictive institution for the mentally ill, with only severely ill patients to relate to. All of these factors lead many potential malingerers to just not bother.

The naive approaches exemplified above have given clinicians clues for developing strategies to detect malingering. The following section describes some of the more commonly used strategies that attempt to expose the signs and symptoms of dissimulation.

DETECTION OF MALINGERING: THE CLINICIAN'S PERSPECTIVE

"The pride of a doctor who has caught a malingerer is akin to that of a fisherman who has landed an enormous fish" (Asher, 1972, p. 145). This quote reflects the adversarial challenge for the clinician faced with a potential malingerer. The task is particularly difficult due to the fact that the clinician can usually only be suspicious that the patient is feigning; "ground truth," or clear evidence of malingering, is seldom available. Thus, the putative "expert" on mental illness must consider the implications for an inaccurate diagnosis. If for example a malingerer is wrongly diagnosed as truly ill, the patient will achieve his/her goals. On the other hand, the false classification of malingering will result in the refusal of medical/psychological care for someone truly in need. This point underscores the difficult experiences some individuals have with the health system when medical "evidence" for their illness is not forthcoming. It is sometimes the case, for example, that individuals with back pain or migraine headaches are accused of malingering (or of having a psychosomatic illness; "it is all in your head"). The clinician must be sensitive to these issues when assessing malingering potential. The shortage of effective tools for detecting malingering furthers the challenge. Nonetheless, there are a number of techniques that aid the clinician.

Clinical Observation

There are a number of signs which, if they are presented frequently, can raise the clinician's suspicion of malingering. For example, one strategy involves looking for *rare symptoms* endorsed by the patient. Such symptoms are rarely reported by bona fide patients. This method was first adopted for use in the Minnesota Multiphasic Personality Inventory (MMPI), a true–false questionnaire commonly used for assessing personality traits (McKinley, Hathaway, & Meehl, 1948). This inventory includes a number of symptoms that are seen in less than 10% of the general population (i.e., the F scale, or "fake bad" index). Thus, if someone endorses a large number of such symptoms, one can suspect that they are over-reporting their difficulties. This strategy has been used effectively with the MMPI and other questionnaires and is based on the "probability" that an average patient will not admit to more than 10% of these rare occurrences.

Another strategy looks for *indiscriminant symptom endorsement.* This approach pays attention to the common tendency of malingerers to believe that "more is better" when reporting problems. Thus, in many cases of feigned illness, individuals will report an unusually large number and variety of symptoms. An impression may be left after a thorough examination that "nobody can be that sick." For example, even in the most severe instances of mental illness, the patient will admit to relatively few psychological symptoms. Therefore, the person that chooses this rather unsophisticated strategy for malingering is usually easily detected. In its extreme form, we have observed that some criminal defendants simulating mental illness may admit to virtually every psychological symptom mentioned by the clinician.

Blatant symptom admission is another potential sign of feigned illness. Many clinical studies suggest that malingerers are more likely to endorse a high percentage of symptoms which are "obvious" indicators of psychopathology. Moreover, one researcher (Greene, 1988) has proposed the use of subtle and obvious scales on the MMPI to detect malingerers. Thus, if the suspected patient endorses a large number of obvious symptoms of illness and ignores more subtle indicators, it may be that he/she is not being truthful. An example would be the case where an individual endorses the obvious signs of schizophrenia—hallucinations, paranoid delusions—but neglects to admit to the lesser known "negative" signs of the disorder such as a disinterest in social relationships, and blunted emotions.

"I frequently hear a Hungarian boys choir singing *Ava Maria* when I eat breakfast." "I am kept awake at night by thoughts that a helicopter will crash through my bedroom window." These complaints are typical examples of *improbable symptoms* occasionally reported by patients. By their preposterous nature, these complaints are never, or very infrequently, reported by either psychiatric patients or healthy people. Thus, individuals who present with such unlikely complaints—particularly if there are several such symptoms—will often be suspected of malingering.

Other clues to malingering are radical inconsistencies in reported symptoms over time, the endorsement of contradictory symptoms (e.g., severe depression and increased appetite), and disparities between reported and observed symptoms (e.g., complaints of tremors but no evidence in interview or ward observations). All of these signs may be useful. The length of stay in the hospital may also be an important a factor in detection, as the longer a clinician may observe the potential malingerer, the greater opportunity to observe contradictions and inconsistencies. Finally, clinicians must also search for corroboration for the reported symptoms from health professionals, family members, and other relevant sources. Of course, this is a well-known and time-honored technique. Many of us have experienced the "doctor's note" requirement to substantiate our reports of illness at school or work.

Structured Interview

Rogers (1988) has discussed the above clinical strategies at length in the literature and has used them as a basis for constructing an interview to detect malingering: *Structured Interview of Reported Symptoms (SIRS)*. In addition to the above techniques, the SIRS is designed to detect unusually large endorsement of symptoms of extreme or "unbearable" severity. An advantage of this structured approach is that it does not rely on the high degree of subjectivity in the idiosyncratic styles of individual clinicians. The approach is more thorough as it applies all of the clinically relevant strategies universally to all patients.

Psychological Tests

A number of psychological tests have been used to detect dissimulation. The widely used MMPI has already been mentioned. This test includes a number of empirically derived strategies for detecting dissimulation and exaggeration (see, e.g., the above discussion of obvious symptoms and "fake bad" strategies). Other "objective" personality tests employ similar scales. In addition, *projective* tests have been used to aid the clinician. The typical example of such a test is the *Rorschach Inkblot Test.* Malingerers on these tests tend to display reduced number of responses, slow reaction times, vague or poor descriptions, dramatic content, and inconsistent responses (Schretlen, 1988). All of these signs may serve to alert the clinician and should not be used by themselves to warrant a classification of malingering. As with all of the above strategies, the clinician must look for frequent and varied signs of malingering and make the judgement based on a thorough evaluation of all information sources.

Other Techniques

Other approaches that have been used have included psychophysiological techniques (Iacono & Patrick, 1988), hypnosis (Miller & Stava, 1988), and drug-assisted inquiry (Rogers & Wettstein, 1988). Psychophysiological techniques, more commonly referred to as "lie detectors," essentially try to contrast the patient's verbal responses to questions with his or her physiological response on a number of measures (e.g., heart rate, sweating, respiratory indices), although their use in detecting malingering is not well-established. Hypnotic techniques have generally been used in cases where patients claim a memory loss to relevant events such as criminal acts. Finally, drug-assisted interviews, better known as "truth serum" strategies, generally employ the use of a barbiturate to place the subject in a more relaxed and less inhibited state. This technique, like hypnosis, attempts to take the potential malingerer "off guard" to elicit a more truthful presentation. Unfortunately, the effectiveness of all of these methods strategies is far from established and, despite their appeal, considerable work needs to be done before they may be applied in a reliable manner.

CONCLUDING COMMENT

The tasks of both the malingerer to feign and the clinician to detect deception are far from simple. The malingerer typically faces a difficult situation in which feigning illness becomes the least unpleasant alternative. As previously outlined, however, the resulting process is complex, as an infinite number of possibilities present themselves to the would-be malingerer. Moreover, in many cases there is little time and few resources to prepare for one's faking. This situation appears to lead many malingerers to take a somewhat naive approach to feigning illness, which in turn enhances the likelihood of their detection.

The task of the clinician is equally demanding. Despite a small body of literature advancing strategies for malingering detection, foolproof techniques to aid the practitioner are not available. The complexity of the task is only accentuated by the negative consequences of an inaccurate determination. As long as a remote possibility of true illness exists, health professionals are understandably reluctant to classify someone as a malingerer. Nonetheless, as health care cutbacks continue to accelerate into the nineties, there is considerable pressure to reserve existing resources for those most deserving. Thus, it is likely that issues of malingering will continue to receive attention by clinicians and researchers alike in order to develop more accurate means for detection.

References

American Psychiatric Association. (1987). *Diagnostic and statistical manual of mental disorders* (3rd ed., revised). Washington, DC: Author.

Asher, R. (1972). *Richard Asher talking sense.* London: University Park Press.

Cleckley, H. (1982). *The mask of sanity* (5th ed.). St. Louis, MO: Mosby.

Greene, R. L. (1988). Assessment of malingering and defensiveness by objective personality measures. In R. Rogers (Ed.), *Clinical assessment of malingering and deception* (pp. 123–158). New York: Guilford.

Hare, R. D. (1991). *The Hare Psychology Checklist—revised.* Toronto: Multi-health Systems.

Hare, R. D., Forth, A. E., & Hart, S. D. (1989). The psychopath as prototype for pathological lying and deception. In J. C. Yuille (Ed.), *Credibility assessment.* New York: Kluwer Academic Publishers.

Hare, R. D., Williamson, S. H., & Harpur, T. J. (1988). Psychopath and language. In T. E. Moffitt & S. A. Mednick (Eds.), *Biological contributions to crime causation* (pp. 68–92). Dordrecht, The Netherlands: Martinus Nijhoff.

Hart, S. D., & Hare, R. D. (1989). Discriminant validity of the psychopathy checklist in a forensic psychiatric population. *Psychological Assessment: A Journal of Consulting and Clinical Psychology, 1,* 211–218.

Iacono, W. G., & Patrick, C. J. (1988) Assessing deception: Polygraph techniques. In R. Rogers (Ed.), *Clinical assessment of malingering and deception* (pp. 205–233). New York: Guilford Press.

Kropp, P. R. & Rogers, R. (1991). *The capacity of psychopaths to malinger.* Unpublished manuscript.

Mckinley, J., Hathaway, S. R., & Meehl, P. E. (1948). The MMPI: K scale. *Journal of Consulting Psychology, 12,* 20–31.

Meadow, R. (1977). Munchausen syndrome by proxy. *Lancet, 2,* 343–345.

Miller, R. D., & Stava, L. J. (1988). Hypnosis and dissimulation. In R. Rogers (Ed.), *Clinical assessment of malingering and deception* (pp. 234–249). New York: Guilford Press.

Roesch, R., & Golding, S. L. (1980). *Competency to stand trial.* Urbana, IL: University of Illinois Press.

Rogers, R. (1988). Structured interviews and dissimulation. In R. Rogers (Ed.), *Clinical assessment of malingering and deception* (pp. 250–268). New York: Guilford Press.

Rogers, R. (1990). Models of feigned mental illness. *Professional Psychology: Research and Practice, 21,* 182–188.

Rogers, R., Bagby, R. M., & Rector, N. (1989). Diagnostic legitimacy of factitious disorder with psychological symptoms. *American Journal of Psychiatry, 146,* 1312–1314.

Rogers, R., Gillis, J. R., & Bagby, R. M. (1990). The SIRS as a measure of malingering: A validation study with a correctional sample. *Behavioral Sciences and the Law, 8,* 85–92.

Rogers, R., & Wettstein, R. M. (1988). Drug-assisted interviews to detect malingering and deception. In R. Rogers (Ed.), *Clinical assessment of malingering and deception* (pp. 195–204). New York: Guilford Press.

Schretlen, D. J. (1988). The use of psychological tests to identify malingered symptoms of a mental disorder. *Clinical Psychological Review, 8,* 451–476.

Sierles, F. S. (1984). Correlates of malingering. *Behavioral Sciences and the Law, 2,* 113–118.

Weighill, V. E. (1983). "Compensation neurosis": A review of the literature. *Journal of Psychosomatic Research, 27,* 97–104.

Index